93656

610.9
Par   Parker, Steve

The history of
medicine

DUE DATE	BRODART	10/93	19.93
MAR 17			
NOV 41			
12-13			
3/10			
10-5-18			
11-1-18			

THE HISTORY OF MEDICINE

Steve Parker

Gareth Stevens Children's Books
MILWAUKEE

93656

For a free color catalog describing Gareth Stevens' list of
high-quality children's books, call 1-800-341-3569 (USA) or
1-800-461-9120 (Canada).

Library of Congress Cataloging-in-Publication Data

Parker, Steve.
    The history of medicine / Steve Parker.
        p. cm. — (Gareth Stevens information library)
    Includes index.
    Summary: Surveys the art and science of medicine from ancient times to the present,
focusing on the most important modern discoveries and innovations in preserving
health, fighting illness, and curing diseases.
    ISBN 0-8368-0024-9
    1. Medicine—History—Juvenile literature. [1. Medicine—History.] I. Title. II. Series.
R133.5.P36 1991
610'.9—dc20   90-23744

North American edition first published in 1992 by
Gareth Stevens Children's Books
1555 North RiverCenter Drive, Suite 201
Milwaukee, Wisconsin 53212, USA

Photographic credits: Ann Ronan Picture Library, 13 (left), 22 (left), 27 (top);
Bibliothèque Nationale, 16; Bodleian Library, 11 (left); Bridgeman Art Library,
4 (center); J. Allan Cash, 32; Mark Edwards, 50 (top); ET Archive, 5, 43 (left);
Format Photographers, 50 (bottom); Giraudon, 25 (bottom); Sally and Richard
Greenhill, 7 (right), 38, 57; Hulton Picture Company, 30 (left), 33 (right);
Hutchinson Library, 47, 48, 51, 52, 53, 54 (right), 56, 58 (left), 59; Imperial War
Museum, 33 (left); The Independent, 58 (right); John Watney Photo Library,
19 (top), 27 (bottom), 30 (bottom), 39 (right), 44 (inset), 45; Magnum, 4 (left),
35 (right), 42, 43 (right); Mansell Collection, 13 (center), 31; Mary Evans Picture
Library, 13 (bottom), 36 (left); Massachusetts General Hospital, 34; Master and
Fellows of Trinity College, Cambridge, 19 (center); National Portrait Gallery,
25 (top); Österreichische National Bibliothek, 17; Peter Newark's Western
Americana, 54 (left); Popperfoto, 7 (left), 35 (top); Queen Mary's Hospital,
Roehampton, 44 (left); Robert Harding Picture Library, 49; Ronald Sheridan's
Picture Library, 12, 13 (top); Science Museum, 10, 11 (right); Science Photo
Library, 32, 37, 39 (left), 40, 41, 43 (top), 44 (bottom); Wellcome Institute, 8, 21,
22 (right); Werner Forman Archive, 55; Windsor Castle, Royal Library, © 1990
Her Majesty the Queen, 20; ZEFA, 4, 9

Illustrated by James Field, Borin van Loon, and Eugene Fleury

Series editors: Neil Champion and Rita Reitci
Research editor: Jennifer Thelen
Educational consultant: Dr. Alistair Ross
Designed by: Groom and Pickerill
Picture research: Ann Usborne
Specialist consultant: Caroline Richmond

Printed in the United States of America

1 2 3 4 5 6 7 8 9 97 96 95 94 93 92

Contents

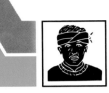

1: HEALTH, ILLNESS, AND MEDICINE

What Is Health? What Is Medicine?

Nuba wrestlers from the Sudan at the peak of fitness. Their life-style and activities involve physical exertion, which keeps the body in good shape. ▼

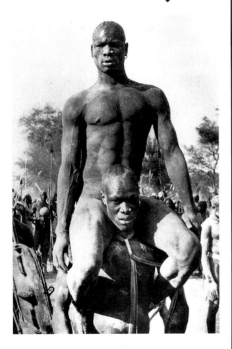

Changing fashions in health. Right: In Queen Elizabeth I's time, it was desirable to be pale. Far right: Today, a suntan is viewed as healthy. But studies show that tanning can be harmful, unless time of exposure is limited and skin and eyes are protected. ▶

Health
Most people have good health for most of the time. But few people enjoy perfect health. Health is more than just the absence of illness. There are always methods of strengthening the body's resistance to disease — for example, by exercising or eating better.

A middle-aged person might seem to be in good health one day. Yet the next day he or she might collapse and die from a heart attack. Another person might seem to be healthy, although bothered by worries. He or she could be deeply depressed, and perhaps even attempt suicide. Good health means both a healthy mind and a healthy body.

Illness
There are many different things in a human body that can go wrong. When a problem

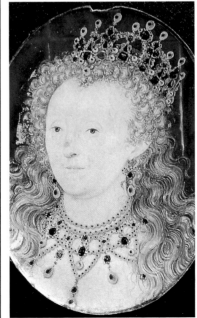

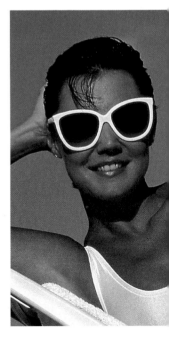

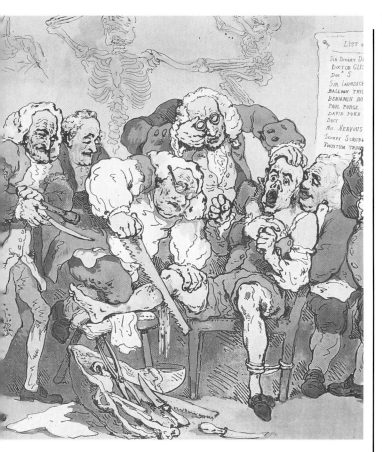

◀ The horrors of amputation, painted by Thomas Rowlandson in 1793. The observers are eager to view the operation and show little interest in the poor patient!

Did You Know?

A few hundred years ago, in many countries, people with mental illnesses were called "mad" and locked away, with no hope of treatment. This still happens in some regions. But recently doctors have begun to understand how the mind works. Now they can treat some kinds of mental illness successfully.

develops, we try to correct it. To get help, we turn to the practice of medicine. Our ideas about health and illness shape our ideas about what we expect from medicine.

Medicine

Doctors and other health workers such as physical and psychiatric therapists, dentists, chiropractors, osteopaths, and nurses provide medical care. They find out what is wrong with us, and try to make us better, or at least to ease our suffering. They treat us with medical drugs, operations, nursing, psychotherapy, and many other forms of care.

It has not always been like this. Through the ages and around the world, people have had very different ideas about health, illness, and medicine. Like science and art, medicine is part of the society and culture we live in. The practice of medicine changes with the times.

WHO's health

In 1948, the United Nations set up an agency called the World Health Organization (WHO). Its aim is the highest possible level of health for all peoples.

WHO's many worldwide medical projects include:

- controlling serious diseases like malaria and tuberculosis

- improving medical services by training doctors and nurses and by providing money to build hospitals and buy drugs and medical equipment

- aiding victims of natural disasters such as famines and earthquakes, since these are times when diseases are more likely to spread

- giving advice to countries on setting up new medical services or on how to improve their existing services.

Staying Healthy

Being responsible

Keeping healthy includes staying in good physical condition, eating the right foods, and avoiding overweight. Not smoking and not drinking too much alcohol also promote good health. Some of these ideas about maintaining health are recent. They may change as we learn more about staying healthy.

People must also check with their doctor about health problems, even small ones, because they might be an early warning sign of something more serious.

▲ Two different practices in taking medicine. Above: In Europe and North America, we simply open a pill bottle and take one of the factory-made tablets. Above right: In rural Sumatra, in Southeast Asia, medicines are carefully prepared from local plants by a recipe handed down through generations.

Handing over responsibility

Some people take little interest in their own bodies. They eat too much and exercise too little. They may smoke or drink to excess. When an illness strikes, they wait until it has become serious before seeing a doctor. Then they expect to be cured. They rely on medicine to take care of them, instead of caring more for themselves.

This attitude has come partly from the success of our modern Western-style medicine. People in places like Europe, North America, and Australia are living longer. We regularly hear about new "wonder" drugs or advances in lifesaving surgery. People may think, Why should I bother to look after myself? Medical care is so good that it will cure me.

The cost of medicine

Modern Western-style medicine cannot cure everyone. There are many diseases, such as certain cancers, that have no cure. Besides, modern medical care is very expensive. Some people cannot afford to pay for it. In countries where health care is run by the state, there are sometimes long waiting lists or shortages of drugs and hospital beds.

It makes more sense to prevent illness instead of treating it after it develops. Medicine is becoming more concerned with prevention. More people want to know how they can look after themselves, and how they can treat their own minor illnesses.

Degrees of illness

- If you go to bed very late one night, you will probably feel tired the next day. You might be absent-minded and slow in your reactions. But most people would not call this being ill. By the day after, you will have recovered.

- If you develop a sore throat and a slight cough, you might be described as slightly ill. You may be able to go on as usual, but with some extra effort for a few days. A century or two ago, you might have been seen as quite healthy if all you had was a slight cough!

- If you catch measles or influenza, you are definitely ill. You will need to be cared for in bed for several days. In this case, a decision has been made that medical care is needed, and you have become a patient.

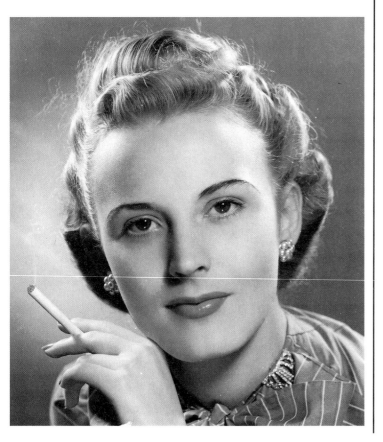

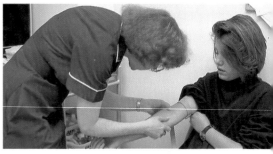

◀ Smoking was once seen as sophisticated or "cool." Today, most people recognize its bad effect on health, and many think of this self-inflicted health hazard as irresponsible.

▲ A blood test helps to reveal early warning signs of disease. It is part of the increasing trend away from treatment and toward prevention.

7

Organizing Medical Care

A Chinese physician talks to his patient and carries out simple tests, such as feeling the quality of the pulse. Every society has its own ideas of what to expect from its medical practitioners. ▶

Spending on health

The United States government spends 4.4% of its total budget on health care. Most of this money goes into childhood illness, diseases such as diabetes, mental illness, to war veterans, and to people who are on Medicare and Medicaid — health insurance plans for people who are old or poor.

A lecture on anatomy during the Middle Ages. Throughout history, training doctors has usually been a long and costly process, from which the public expects good care. ▶

In the past, there was little scientific knowledge about the human body and the causes of its ailments. This was also a time when few people had any interest in researching the cause and cure of disease. Although most doctors knew little science, they still tried to care for whatever illnesses they encountered. Just as medical knowledge has expanded, so has health care gone far beyond the efforts of any one doctor.

Levels of care

Medical services are organized into several levels. No single doctor is an expert in all

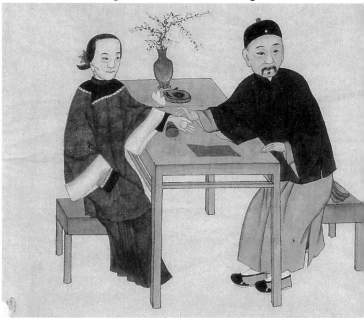

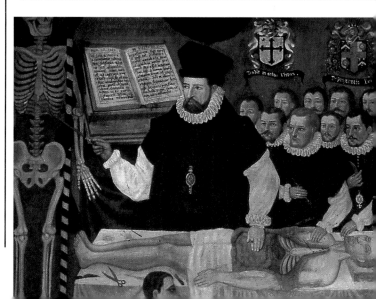

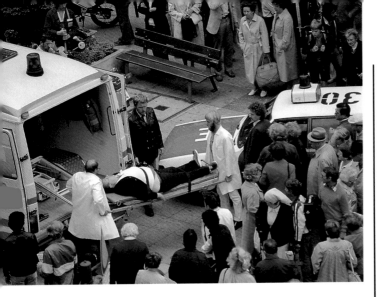

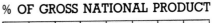
◀ Emergency care from a fully trained ambulance staff.

areas of medicine, nor can a single doctor afford all the medical equipment that is used in today's treatments. So we concentrate skills and facilities in specialists and hospitals.

Primary care

The primary care level involves the family doctor, often called a general practitioner. He or she is the first person we are likely to see when we become ill. The family doctor works in a local area and can identify and treat common illnesses.

Secondary care

The secondary care level involves hospitals and specialists. In serious cases, the family doctor sends the patient to a specialist or to a hospital for tests and treatments.

The hospital has specialized doctors and nurses. Some concentrate on certain parts of the body. For example, a cardiologist treats heart problems, and an orthopedic surgeon deals with bones and muscles. Other doctors specialize in health problems that people encounter at a certain stage of life. For instance, pediatricians care for children, and obstetricians look after pregnant women and their developing babies.

Other hospital staff members include laboratory technicians, who test blood and urine, and technicians who operate special types of equipment, such as x-ray machines.

% **OF GROSS NATIONAL PRODUCT**

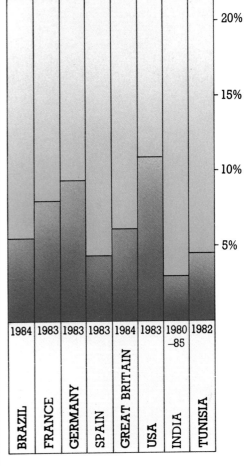

1984	1983	1983	1983	1984	1983	1980–85	1982
BRAZIL	FRANCE	GERMANY	SPAIN	GREAT BRITAIN	USA	INDIA	TUNISIA

▲ Percentages of gross national product spent on health care by selected countries in a recent year.

9

MEDICINE IN ANCIENT TIMES

The Beginnings of Medicine

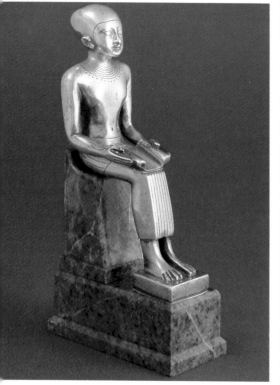

▲ A statue of Imhotep, an early doctor. Ancient Egyptians worshiped him as a god.

This carved stone relief on the wall of an ancient Egyptian temple shows some of the surgical instruments in use at the time, including pincers and saws. ▶

Humans live together in groups and help one another. They share food, look after children, and try to help those who fall ill. This is how medicine began. Some people became more skilled at healing than others. They took on the role of looking after the sick, and became the first doctors.

Long before people wrote history, we have evidence of medical care. The skeletons of some Neanderthal people had bones that were so deformed that when alive they would not have been able to feed or take care of themselves. Others must have cared for them.

Other skeletons from ancient burial grounds show signs of broken bones that had been set. Someone had positioned the broken parts so that they would grow back together correctly and heal well.

Trepanning

Clear signs of the first medical operations are neat holes in skulls, some of them over 10,000 years old. The holes resulted from a process called trepanning. This was first carried out

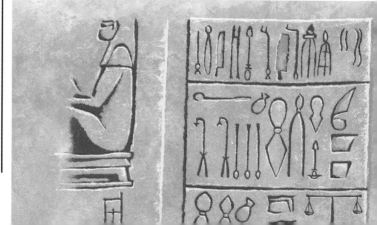

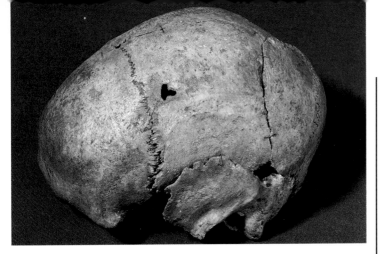

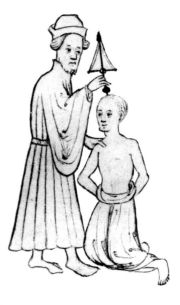

using stone cutters or scrapers to gouge through the skin, the muscle, and then bone to the brain beneath. This may have been part of a magical ritual to release evil spirits inside the head of the patient.

In ancient Egypt

About 4,600 years ago, Imhotep lived in ancient Egypt. He was a court architect, sculptor, and doctor. People traveled from far and wide to be treated by him. After he died, his people made him into a god. The sick flocked to his temples and worshiped statues of him in the hope of being cured.

The ancient Egyptians believed that each part of the body was watched over by a god. If disease developed in that part, they thought that prayers, offerings, and sacrifices to that god might bring about a cure. They also used medicines. They put moldy bread on wounds — and we now know a type of bread mold produces the antibiotic drug penicillin. They also used poppy sap, which contains pain-deadening opium, to relieve suffering.

Ancient modern medicine

Two papyrus documents from about 3,500 years ago contain descriptions of the medical techniques of ancient Egypt.

The Smith papyrus tells how to set broken bones, how the pulse in the wrist can show the health of the heart, how to treat eye disease, how to stop bleeding by pressing on the wound, and many other procedures. Some are still in use today. This papyrus may be a copy of an earlier version, perhaps 1,000 years older.

The Ebers papyrus discusses about 900 medications, such as tannic acid for burns and castor oil as a cure for constipation. It also gives chants and prayers to the gods for specific illnesses. The god of physicians was Thoth, of whom the Ebers papyrus says, "He gives to the physicians skill to cure."

This papyrus also shows that the ancient physicians prescribed special diets, massages, and hypnosis for their patients.

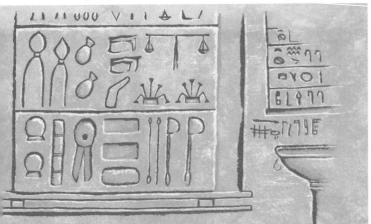

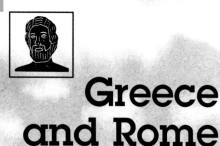

Greece and Rome

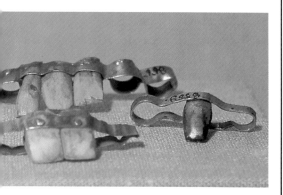

▲ The Roman hospitals, called *valetudinaria*, were clean and well-ordered places, where ill citizens and injured soldiers could rest and recover.

▲ False teeth from ancient Rome, set in a gold bridge. Dental care was only one branch of the complex Roman health care system.

The Greeks

For 800 years, from 2,600 to 1,800 years ago, the ancient Greeks had a complex system of medical care.

Alcmaeon (born about 535 BC) is one of the first people known to have dissected — cut open and studied — the bodies of dead people for medical purposes.

Empedocles (born about 492 BC) saw that the heart was connected into the network of blood vessels.

Aristotle (born about 384 BC) studied and dissected many animals. He held a firm belief in the scientific method of making careful observations, doing experiments, and noting causes and their effects.

Roman advances

In the first century AD, Celsus wrote *De Medicina*, a medical encyclopedia in eight volumes that showed the state of Roman medicine. Doctors were taught and paid by the state. The Romans began the first true hospitals, open to the general public. They built canals and aqueducts to supply fresh, clean water. They disposed of sewage properly. Both dirty water and poor sewage disposal encourage disease.

The great Galen

Galen (born about AD 130) was a Greek who settled in Rome. He spent time dissecting animals, including monkeys, and applied his observations to the human body. He wrote hundreds of books describing the skeleton, muscles, and nerves, the brain, and the workings of the spinal cord. His teachings form the basis of the part of medicine known as anatomy. This is the study of the structure of the human body and its many organs.

Galen was a physician and anatomist. His many books summarized the medical knowledge of the day. After his time, and with the breakdown of the Roman Empire, medicine entered the Dark Ages. Little progress was made for several centuries.

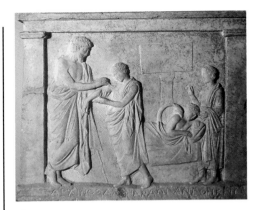

▲ Asklepios treating a patient in the fourth century BC. Temples were built in his honor, where people visited and prayed to be healed.

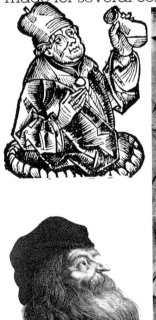
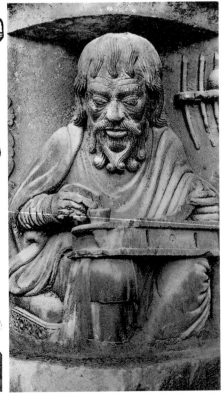

Dreams and illness

Like the Egyptians, the Greeks mixed medicine with religion, magic, and superstition. Many of the physicians worshiped Asklepios, a doctor whom they had made into a god — later called Aesculapius by the Romans. The patient came to one of the temples dedicated to him, and slept there overnight. In the morning, he or she described any dreams to a priest, who interpreted their meaning and prescribed treatment.

◀ Far left, top: Galen was a great physician and one of the chief founders of the science of anatomy. But his errors went unchallenged for centuries. Far left, bottom: Empedocles, a philosopher from ancient Greece, studied the heart and blood vessels. Left: Aristotle was the chief founder of comparative anatomy, which describes and compares the parts of animals. But it is doubtful that he studied the insides of human corpses.

13

The Father of Medicine

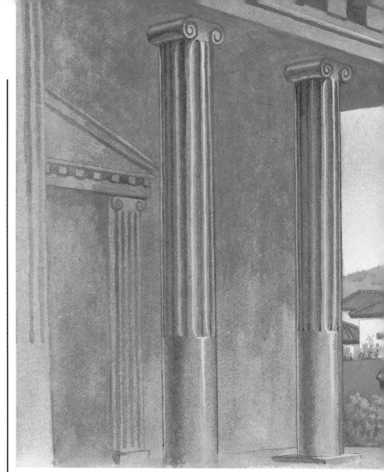

Hippocrates of Cos was a doctor and surgeon of Greece. He was born about 460 BC and spent many years in his birthplace, the Greek island of Cos, in charge of the medical school and hospital there. His writings and teachings, and those of his fellow teachers and students, helped to form the basis of modern medicine.

Hippocratic teachings

In ancient Greece, medicine was bound up with religion and magic. Hippocrates and the other teaching physicians tried to encourage a simple and sensible approach that did not involve spirits and the supernatural world.

They taught that the doctor should examine the patient carefully and try to identify, or diagnose, the illness from the condition of the patient, not from stories that others had told or religious "signs." The doctor was also taught to look for causes of disease in the environment, in food or drink, or in the workplace, and give advice on prevention.

Medicine's founders

Hippocrates is often called the Father of Medicine. But no one person was medicine's founder. Many other Greeks and Romans helped to establish medicine as a systematic discipline.

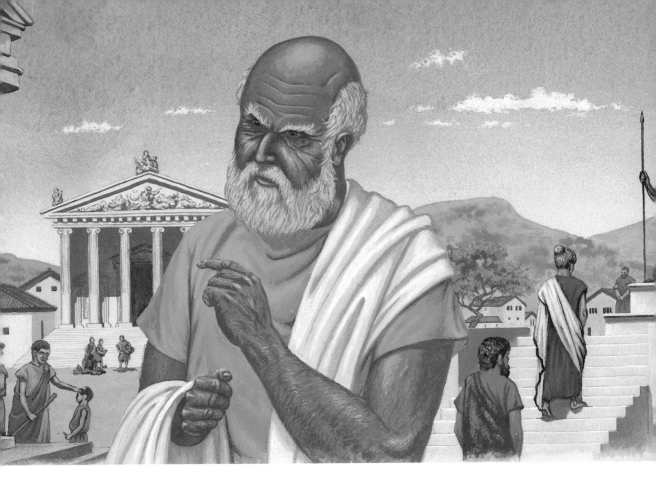

The doctor should give treatment only when necessary. Hippocrates recognized rightly that the body has amazing powers to heal itself of less serious illnesses. Unnecessary treatment could interfere with this healing. He taught that treatment should be as simple as possible, such as a change in food. The doctor should observe the effect of the treatment and keep records of the patient's case. Later, the doctor should study the records and learn from them.

A moral code for medicine

Hippocrates and his colleagues devised guidelines about how doctors should think and behave. They wrote that a doctor's main aim is to help the patient, not to become rich or famous. Doctors should be sensible, thoughtful, well-trained, clean, and modest. When a doctor obtains personal information about a patient, this should not be told to others. This is called the principle of confidentiality, and is still followed today.

▲ Hippocrates as he might have walked through the medical school and hospital on Cos. Besides teaching medicine, he encouraged good hygiene and high standards of moral and professional behavior among doctors.

Elements and humors

Many scholars of ancient times, including Aristotle, believed in the four "qualities" of life: hot, cold, wet, and dry. These combined with four "elements": earth, air, fire, and water. If the combinations in the body were unbalanced, illness resulted. Later, illness was linked to imbalance of the four body "humors," or liquids: phlegm, blood, yellow bile, and black bile. These ideas lasted for many centuries.

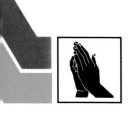

3: MEDIEVAL MEDICINE

Advances under Islam

In Europe, the Middle Ages lasted from the fifth to about the fourteenth centuries. During this period, there was little progress in any science, including medicine. The skills of the Egyptians, Greeks, and the Romans were forgotten.

But in other parts of the world, medical knowledge was growing. The knowledge of the Greeks had been translated into Arabic, the language of Islam. As the Islamic empire grew in the seventh century, its physicians developed this medical knowledge further.

The Black Death

The Black Death, or bubonic plague, is a disease caused by bacteria. It has killed many millions of people throughout history. It is spread by the bites of fleas that have sucked blood from infected rats, and by droplets coughed up or sneezed out by people.

The Black Death swept across Europe and western Asia from AD 551 to 555. In Constantinople, the disease killed 10,000 people every day.

In 1346-50, bubonic plague killed 25 million people in Europe. It was called the Black Death partly because bleeding in the skin made dark patches.

Doctors of the time could not halt the spread of bubonic plague. Today we can prevent its spread because we know it is carried by fleas. It can now be cured if antibiotics are given without delay.

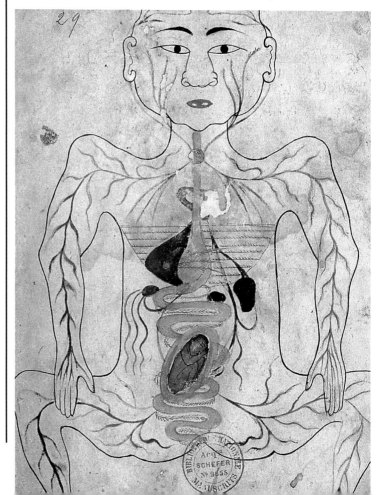

A drawing of a pregnant woman showing the heart, blood vessels, and other internal organs. This picture was prepared for a Persian prince during the tenth century. ▶

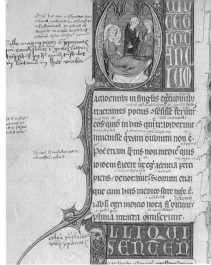

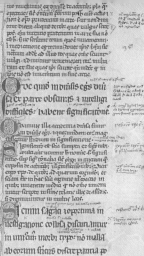

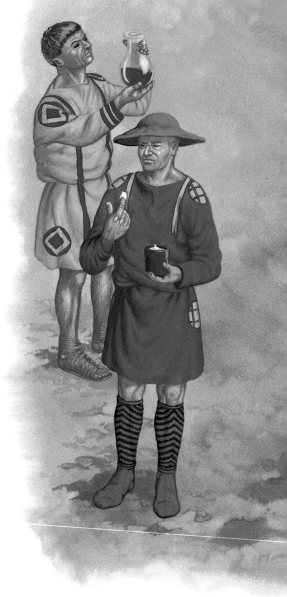

This is a page from an Arabic medical text translated into Latin, the language spoken by educated people in Europe. Arabic medical works were used in European medical schools.

Famous Persian physicians

In Persia, now Iran, a famous doctor known as Rhazes lived until AD 923. He gave one of the first descriptions of measles. He also wrote many medical books, including the enormous encyclopedia *Kitab al-hawi*.

The Persian physicians were skilled at inventing and using new drugs. In fact, our words *drug* and *alcohol* have Arabic origins. In AD 977, a hospital was set up in Baghdad. Here, over 20 doctors carried out operations and ran a clinic for eye diseases.

In the early eleventh century, the Persian philosopher Ibn Sina, also known as Avicenna, practiced medicine and wrote many medical books. His great encyclopedia, *Canon of Medicine*, was based on Greek and Roman works. It was translated into other languages, including Latin, and became an important text in European medical schools for the next several centuries.

Progress in India

Farther east, new medical knowledge emerged. In India, during the fifth century, the great physician Susruta could choose from over 100 surgical instruments for operations and over 700 medicinal plants for drug treatments. He rightly believed that mosquitoes spread malaria and rats spread bubonic plague. The doctors of his time could set broken bones, if the skin was still intact.

Cosmas and Damian, two saints famous for healing. Many saints were credited with healing abilities, especially from the fourth to sixth centuries.

Mixing Medicine and Religion

Monks pray for the souls of sick people in a medieval sanitarium. By asking for forgiveness and help from spiritual powers, they hoped to aid the healing of their patients. ▼

Throughout history, in various parts of the world, medicine has been linked with religion. Changes in religious beliefs have affected medical knowledge, and the reverse has also happened. As Christianity gradually replaced native beliefs by about the twelfth century, it also changed the practice of medicine.

Body and soul

The Christian teachings of concern for others and helping the feeble and sick led to the founding of hospitals and care centers for the poor. These were often run by monks, partly because they were among the few people who could read. Medical works, especially those of Aristotle and Galen, were in Latin, the language of European scholars at that time.

During this period, Christianity viewed illness as being caused by spirits or supernatural events, such as "punishment from God" or a "visit of the Devil." While herbs and medicines were used in treatment, prayers and offerings made to cleanse the soul were common. The

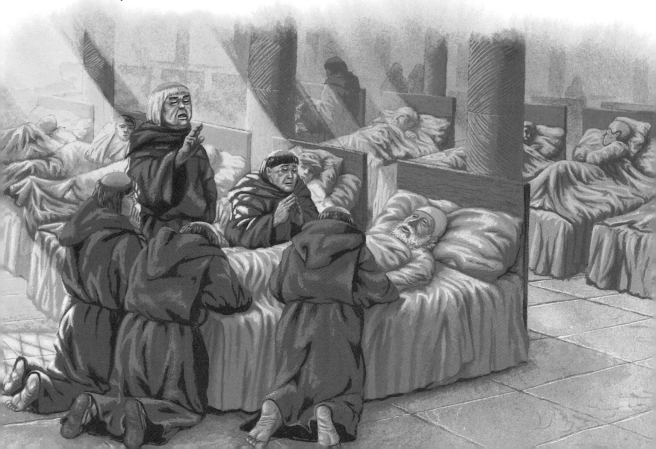

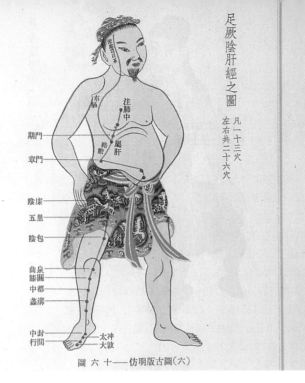

足厥陰肝經之圖

凡一十三穴
左右共二十六穴

期門

章門

陰廉
五里
陰包

曲泉
膝關
中都
蠡溝

中封
行間
太冲
大敦

圖十六——仿明版古圖（六）

workings of the physical body and its ailments were seen as less important. For a long time, it was forbidden, for religious reasons, to dissect a corpse for the purpose of medical study.

As a result, what we today call scientific medicine hardly progressed. The knowledge of Galen and other Greeks and the Romans was followed, but in time it became confused and mixed with magic and superstition.

Eastern progress

During the Dark Ages in Europe, medicine was developing in other regions, such as India. In China, in about AD 620-30, Chen Ch'uan was probably the first physician to notice the typical symptoms of diabetes. Starting in the sixth century, the Chinese spent ten centuries in compiling a vast encyclopedia. This huge work described more than 1,000 drugs.

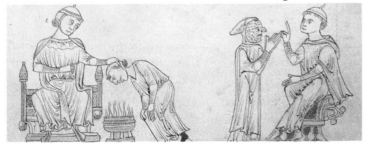

◀ A chart of acupuncture points used in Eastern medicine. This system is based on balancing the body's flow of energy.

The doctrine of signatures

Many myths have arisen about the healing powers of plants. Some became included in the doctrine of signatures. This doctrine says that if a plant resembles a part of the human body, it can be used to cure that part of an illness. For example, the flowers of eyebright have a blotchy, bloodshot appearance — and so they were prescribed for red, sore eyes. Lungwort leaves are rounded, with white speckles — and so they were advised for lung diseases. The root of meadow saffron looks like a foot swollen with gout — and so it should treat this condition. There was often some truth in these beliefs. Meadow saffron root is rich in colchicine, a chemical used to treat gout.

This ginseng root looks like the legs of a human. Plant parts that resembled body parts formed the basis for the doctrine of signatures. ▼

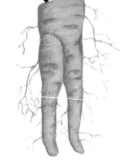

◀ Physicians and patients in a thirteenth-century work from Salerno. Heat therapy is shown on the left. A person with leprosy is on the right.

Studying Body Structure

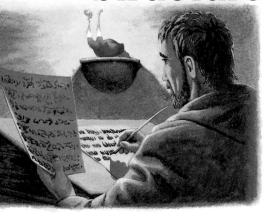

In the third century BC, a Chinese medical book called *Medicine of the Yellow Emperor* described human anatomy. But Western medicine paid little attention to anatomy.

In the ninth century, in Salerno, Italy, a medical school was established for teaching men and women doctors and for treating patients. The Salerno medical students studied anatomy and took examinations after five years. By the twelfth century, the Salerno medical school was famous throughout Europe and Asia. Slowly it became less prominent as other centers of learning were established in places like Bologna, Italy, and later in Montpellier, France.

Renaissance medicine

The Renaissance period began in northern Italy during the early fourteenth century. There was a rapid rebirth of the sciences and the arts from their classical beginnings many centuries before the Dark Ages. Painting, sculpture, architecture, and music made great progress. So did medicine.

▲ Constantine of Carthage translated Arabic medical works into Latin at the Salerno medical school in around 1050-80. Latin was the language used in European schools at the time.

Art and anatomy

Leonardo da Vinci lived from 1452 to 1519. His genius for both art and science led him to state openly that Galen could be wrong. But Leonardo's detailed anatomical drawings of humans and animals and his many experiments were not published at the time. They made little impact on medical progress.

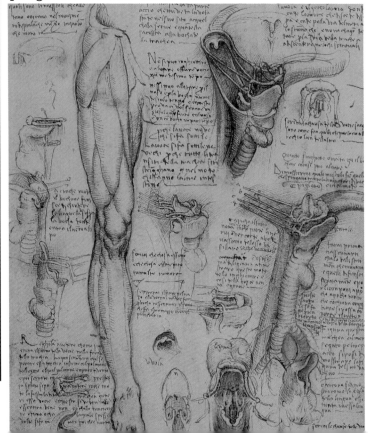

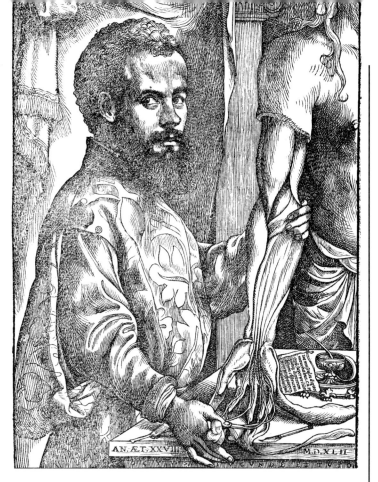

◀ Andreas Vesalius, professor of anatomy at Padua, dissects the arm muscles.

The Padua school

After Vesalius, the Padua medical school produced many more skilled physicians and anatomists:

- In the 1500s, Gabriello Fallopio studied many parts of the body in minute detail. The fallopian tubes in the female body are named after him.

- Santorio Sanctorius (1561-1636) began the study of body chemistry and helped found the science of physiology. He made devices to measure body pulse and temperature.

Great artists of the period such as Michelangelo and Leonardo da Vinci studied the human form closely. Some of them dissected human and animal bodies and studied the muscles and organs to make their drawings more accurate.

The work of Vesalius

During the 1530s, Andreas Vesalius, a medical student from Brussels, saw the need to replace Galen's works with a more accurate version. He went to the medical school in Padua, Italy, where he became professor of anatomy and surgery in 1538.

In 1543, Vesalius published his momentous book *De Humani Corporis Fabrica*. He pointed out and corrected many of Galen's mistakes. Vesalius showed that in order to treat the body when ill, doctors needed to understand the structure and workings of the body when it is healthy. Upon this foundation, medicine entered a new era.

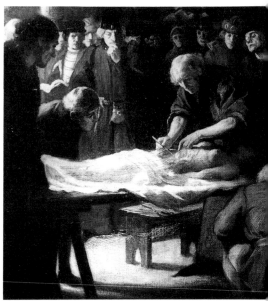

▲ Mondino dei Liucci carries out a dissection at Bologna in 1318. He reintroduced anatomy into medical school teaching.

◀◀ Opposite: Detailed anatomical sketches from one of Leonardo da Vinci's notebooks.

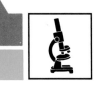

4: SCIENTIFIC BEGINNINGS

Experiment and Observation

During the sixteenth century, the pace of medical progress increased in Europe. The printing press made books more widely available, so researchers and doctors could share and learn from each other's work. The Renaissance inspired a desire for new scientific knowledge. Later, the Industrial Revolution allowed mass production of medical machines and equipment.

Only some medicine before this time had been scientific. It was based on careful observation, looking at causes and effects, developing theories about why things happen, and using experiments to test the theories. But now scientific methods were being used more widely, and with greater attention to detail.

Fernel and Paracelsus

Understanding of the body's anatomy and physiology was increasing all the time. Soon physicians began to apply this knowledge to

Occupational diseases

Paracelsus recognized that a person's job could cause illness, for example, miner's lung. Later, in the seventeenth century, Bernardino Ramazzini, an Italian physician, listed 40 jobs and trades, together with the illnesses linked to them, such as cancers. Ramazzini was professor of medicine at Modena, Padua, and then Venice. His work set the foundation for the study of occupational medicine.

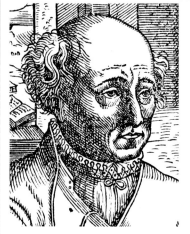 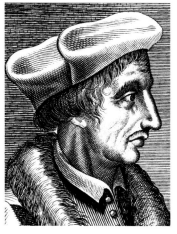

Right: Paracelsus (1493-1541), as portrayed in his work *Astronomica et astrologica* (1567). Far right: Jean Fernel (1506-88), shown in a line engraving published in 1682. ▶

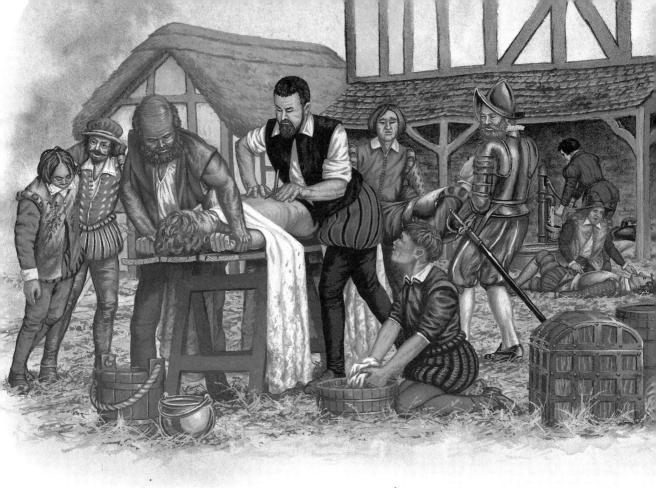

diseases and their treatments. Jean François Fernel was professor of medicine at Paris. His textbook of 1554, *Universa Medicina*, broke new ground. The first part describes human physiology and anatomy. The second part deals with pathology — the study of human organs in their diseased state. The third part of the book discusses treatments.

Around this time, the renowned Paracelsus was traveling in Europe and treating patients. In 1526 he became professor at the University of Basel in Switzerland. Paracelsus introduced new chemical drugs, such as those containing mercury, sulfur, antimony, lead, iron, and copper. He also encouraged his patients to talk about their illness. This was a teaching of Hippocrates, but one which many physicians had forgotten. Paracelsus also had faith in the healing power of nature. Instead of the complicated prescriptions of the time, he advised simple dressings for wounds and giving drugs one at a time and judging the result of each.

▲ Ambroise (Andre) Paré was a leading French army surgeon from 1536 to 1545 and then surgeon-in-chief to four French kings in succession.

Infectious diseases

Over the centuries, physicians had vague ideas about germs as the causes of certain diseases. In 1546, Italian physician Girolamo Fracastoro published a book describing diseases that could be spread from person to person by "minute bodies." He mentions three ways of spreading: by touching parts of the ill person's body; by touching an object already touched by the ill person; and by being in the same place as the ill person. Fracastoro suspected that tiny germs existed, but there were no microscopes as yet, so he could not prove his theories.

Medical Advances

▲ William Harvey applied the principles of hydraulics to his discovery of how the heart circulates blood. At the time, many new machines were being developed, with pumps and tubes and flowing liquids, and these may have inspired Harvey in his reasoning.

Opposite, top: Thomas Sydenham advanced the art of diagnosis. Opposite, bottom: Pierre Fauchard helped to establish dentistry. ▶ ▶

In 1628, English physician William Harvey published a book called *An Anatomical Discussion on the Movement of the Heart and Blood in Animals.*

Until Harvey's time, most physicians followed the old teachings of Galen. The heart was said to warm the blood, which was made in the liver and seeped from veins to arteries through little holes in the heart's dividing wall. The heartbeat and pulse were the result of the blood ebbing to and fro in the blood vessels, as it was enriched by a "vital spirit."

The Italian anatomists showed that blood could not seep through the heart's central wall, but they could not explain what happened instead. Harvey figured out that blood must flow continuously around the body in one direction only, with the heart as the pump. This discovery had far-reaching effects on all fields of medicine.

24

Over the next two centuries, there were many momentous medical advances in Europe. People in other parts of the world had already made some of these discoveries, in certain cases centuries before. But many of their findings had not led to further progress. The European advances are important because they were steps that led to the scientific Western-style medicine we use today.

William Harvey
During his research, Harvey saw that the valves in the blood vessels resembled the valves being designed into hydraulic machines at the time to control the flow of liquids. In a similar way, the valves of the heart and the blood vessels kept the blood moving in one direction as it was pushed by the heart. But Harvey could not say how blood got from the small arteries to small veins.

Thomas Sydenham
Thomas Sydenham has been called the "English Hippocrates," and he had similarities with the great Greek physician. He was the first to describe scarlet fever. Sydenham emphasized the need to diagnose diseases correctly, and how to observe, care for, and treat patients. He used cinchona bark, which contains the drug quinine, to treat malaria. He gave iron for anemia, and prescribed opium to deaden great pain. In 1666, he published *The Method of Treating Fevers*. Sydenham believed that doctors should help guide the body's own healing powers, and his notes on the case histories of patients are still admired today.

Pierre Fauchard
Chinese specialists had been filling and capping teeth with gold for many centuries. French surgeon Pierre Fauchard introduced the idea of dentistry as a medical specialty. In 1728 he published *The Surgeon Dentist, or Treatise of the Teeth*.

Did You Know?

Taking a person's pulse was not always the common routine that it is today. John Floyer, an English doctor, was one of the first Europeans to suggest that the pulse rate could be used to assess a patient's health. In 1707, he described his method, and he even proposed a special watch to make accurate counts.

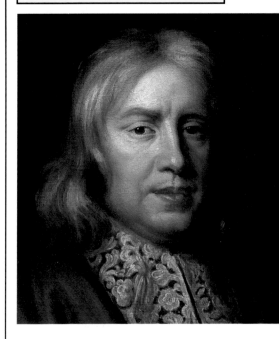

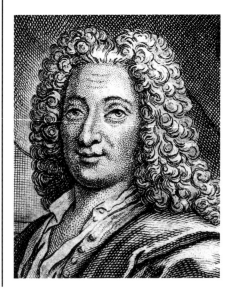

Medicine Branches Out

Edward Jenner

Edward Jenner was an English country doctor who developed the idea of vaccination. At that time, smallpox was a serious and often fatal disease. Jenner knew of the popular belief that people who had cowpox, a mild form of smallpox caught from cattle, would not later get smallpox. In 1796, he inoculated a boy, James Phipps, with cowpox. He did this by putting into the boy's skin fluid from the sores of a dairymaid who had cowpox. Weeks later, he inoculated Phipps with smallpox. The boy did not develop the disease. Vaccination, also called inoculation, has since saved numerous people from this and other diseases.

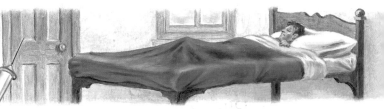

Thomas Hodgkin

In the early 1800s, Thomas Hodgkin became a physician at Guy's Hospital, London. His interest was pathology, the study of how the body parts respond and change during disease. Hodgkin helped to make the pathologist an important member of the medical team. The work of this specialist had practical value in treating illness, as well as being of purely scientific interest.

Louis Pasteur

Louis Pasteur was a chemist and professor at Lille and Paris. In the mid-1800s, he showed that changes such as the fermenting of beer and the souring of milk were caused by tiny organisms that floated on the dust in the air or were carried on objects. He devised a method of keeping wine from spoiling by heating it to a certain temperature and so killing any microbes it may have had. Today, we pasteurize milk and other foods to make them safe to eat.

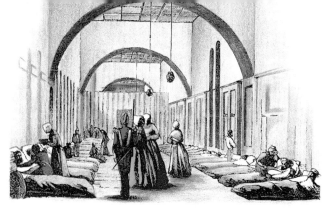

Florence Nightingale

In the mid-1800s, Englishwoman Florence Nightingale traveled to the Crimea and Turkey to help care for wounded British soldiers who were fighting there. Her dedication and skill soon led to new nursing methods. On her return to London in 1860, she began the world's first training school for nurses, with high standards for food, hygiene, and health care in bright, clean, airy wards. She is the founder of the modern nursing profession.

Joseph Lister

Since the Renaissance, surgical techniques had been improving. But the infections that wounds brought still killed many patients. During the mid-1800s, Joseph Lister was a professor of surgery at Glasgow, Edinburgh, and then London. He expanded Pasteur's work and tried to prevent microbes from infecting patients with chemicals called antiseptics, which killed the organisms. Surgery soon became much safer.

Robert Koch

In the late 1800s, a German physician, Robert Koch, established the branch of medicine known as bacteriology. He continued the work of Pasteur and showed that certain types of microbes, especially bacteria, are the cause of many infectious diseases. He studied anthrax, and in 1882, he discovered Koch's bacillus, the bacterium that causes the widespread and often fatal disease tuberculosis. He also developed ways of grouping and naming bacteria and growing them under standard culture conditions in the laboratory.

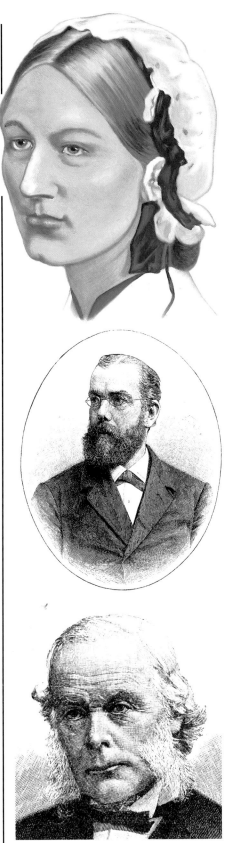

Microscopes and Medicine

In 1628, the same year that William Harvey published his great work, Marcello Malpighi was born in Italy. He became a professor at Pisa and Bologna. He was the first anatomist to use a microscope.

Galileo had made an early type of microscope in the 1500s. Malpighi used a better version to study body tissues such as liver, skin, and bone. In 1661, while examining a frog's lung, he saw the capillaries that connect arteries and veins, so completing the blood circuit first explored by Harvey. Malpighi discovered the taste buds of the tongue. He also studied the development of eggs, helping to establish the science of embryology.

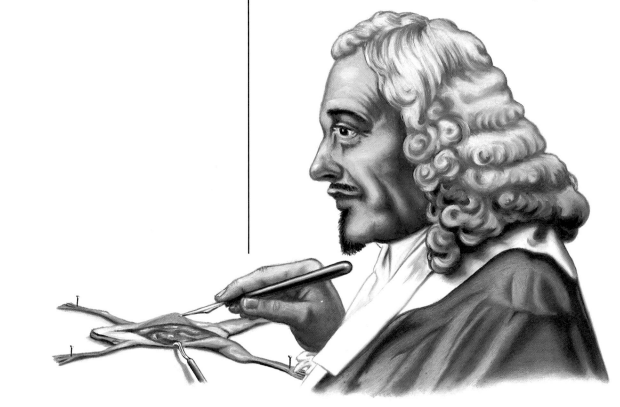

▲ Marcello Malpighi studies the microscopic structure of frog tissues. Malpighian tubules in insects and malpighian bodies in mammals' kidneys are named after him. These structures help rid the body of wastes.

The draper of Delft

Around the same time, Anton van Leeuwenhoek was peering through a simple homemade microscope of his own design. A draper, or fabric and clothing dealer, from Delft, Holland, he had no scientific training. Yet he ground his own lenses and saw and

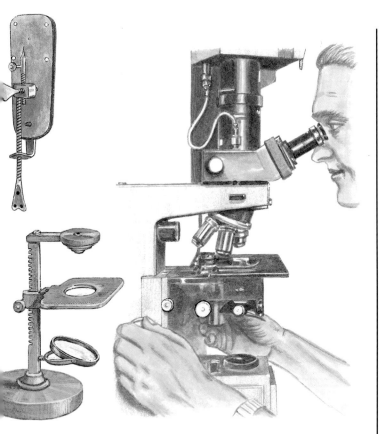

◀ Far left, top: Leeuwenhoek's first microscope, a hand-held model just over three inches (8 cm) high. Far left, bottom: A later model by Leeuwenhoek could stand on a table. Left: A modern electron microscope that can see details of structures inside cells.

described red blood cells, muscle fibers, and the sperm from the male sex organs. In 1683, he drew diagrams of harmless bacteria from his own mouth.

In time, medicine adopted the microscope to help in diagnosis — discovering the causes and effects of disease. In the late 1800s, improvements in microscope equipment began a new era in microscopic medicine.

The cell theory

In the first half of the nineteenth century, biologists were developing the theory that all living things are composed of tiny units that they called cells. Medicine began to apply this knowledge to the human body.

Jakob Henle studied many human organs under the microscope and helped to show that they were indeed made of cells. In the 1800s, he unraveled the microstructure of the kidney. He also studied the eye, the brain, and the muscles in the walls of arteries.

Cellular pathology

Rudolf Virchow was a Prussian statesman, anthropologist, and pathologist. Like Henle, he showed that body tissues were composed of cells and their products. Virchow proposed that every cell in the body had been produced from a cell. This process could be traced back through the body's development to a single first cell — the fertilized egg.

Virchow extended his work into medicine by showing that diseases are the result of cells working incorrectly or being destroyed. These changes could be seen through the microscope. His ideas led to the founding of the branch of medicine known as cellular pathology. Today, this is a vital part of the study and treatment of many diseases, such as cancers.

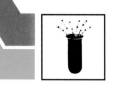

5: | A TIME OF RAPID PROGRESS

The Era of Drugs

Frederick Banting and Charles Best, with the first dog they injected with insulin, in 1921. These men developed the first treatment for the condition of diabetes — by using the hormone insulin. ▼

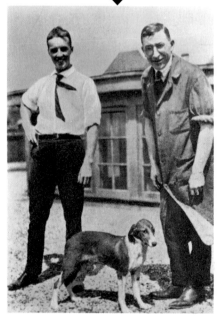

In 1900, the American military surgeon Walter Reed led a team that showed that the disease yellow fever was spread by the bite of a certain mosquito, *Aedes aegypti*. The following year, Reed identified the virus responsible. Within a few years, the areas where the disease lurked was greatly reduced by clearing mosquito-breeding zones in southern North America, Central and South America, and parts of Africa.

Also in 1900, Scottish military officer William Leishman discovered that the tropical disease kala-azar was spread by sand flies. It was caused by a tiny one-celled animal parasite that multiplied in the blood. We now know this disease as leishmaniasis.

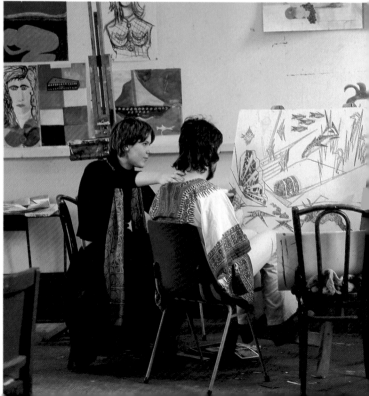

This psychiatric patient is being helped by art therapy, where painting and drawing are an aid to recovery. Many new forms of therapy developed as psychiatric medicine progressed. ▶

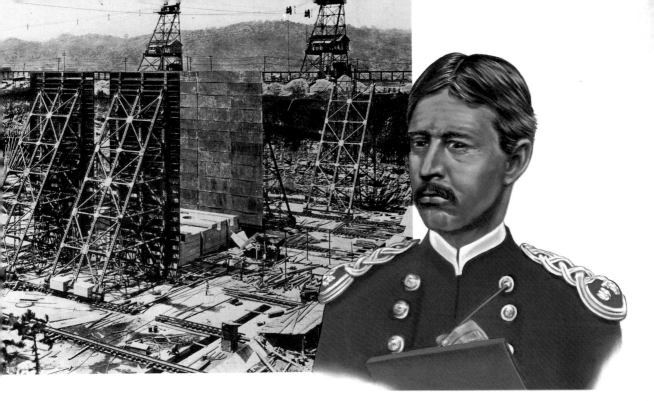

▲ Walter Reed makes medical notes at his "battleground" against yellow fever, the Panama Canal construction site.

Blood groups

In 1900, Austrian scientist and doctor Karl Landsteiner showed that not all human blood was the same. He found at least three groups — A, B, and O. Soon after, he identified the AB group. Landsteiner also unraveled the Rhesus, or Rh, blood types, in about 1940. This pioneering work of blood grouping and typing made blood transfusions and surgery immensely safer.

Mental illness

In 1900, Sigmund Freud, a Viennese physician, published his work *The Interpretation of Dreams*. Freud established the basic principles of psychiatry.

Patterns of progress

During the early 1900s, the pattern of progress gradually changed. Medical research became more complex and expensive. The era of the lone pioneering doctor, making far-reaching discoveries in a home laboratory, was ending. Teams of researchers, using sophisticated equipment, laboratories, and hospital facilities, became more common.

Modern drug therapy

In 1908, German bacteriologist Paul Ehrlich won the Nobel Prize for medicine. Ehrlich had studied the process of immunity — the way the body develops resistance to certain infections after it has suffered from them once. Working with Emil von Behring, he developed an immunization method for the children's disease diphtheria.

In 1910, Ehrlich introduced the laboratory-made drug Salvarsan (arsphenamine) to treat the disease syphilis. This was the beginning of modern drug therapy, where new drugs are made chemically, rather than being extracted from plants or animals.

31

Antibiotics, the Wonder Drugs

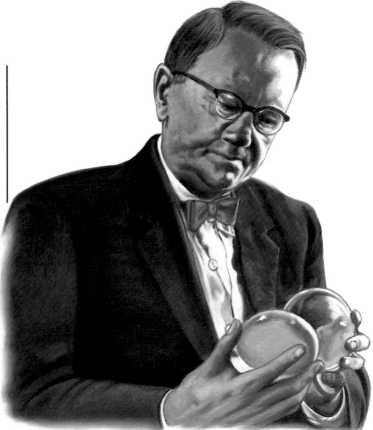

Alexander Fleming checks the growth of bacteria on a culture plate that has been inoculated with penicillin. ▶

Tropical swamps like this one are breeding grounds for the *Anopheles* mosquito, whose bite can spread malaria. ▼

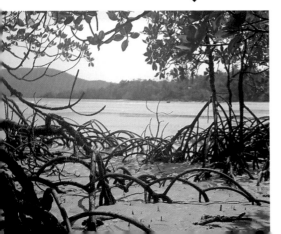

In 1928, an accident sparked one of the greatest advances in medicine.

British scientist Alexander Fleming was studying bacteria in his laboratory. He used the standard technique of growing the bacteria on nutrient jelly in small round culture plates. Somehow, airborne spores of a mold contaminated one plate. As the mold grew, Fleming noticed that nearby bacteria died.

Fleming began working with this effect. He found that a substance produced by the mold could kill several types of bacteria that caused common infections. The mold's scientific name was *Penicillium notatum*, and so Fleming called this new substance penicillin.

Large-scale production and testing

The next task was to make pure penicillin in large quantities for tests on people. University of Oxford scientists Howard Florey and Ernst Chain achieved this. The first tests, run during the Second World War, were highly successful. This was the beginning of the era of antibiotic drugs, which are often called wonder drugs.

In 1943, American microbiologist Selman Waksman discovered streptomycin, another powerful antibiotic made by a mold that grows in soil. Waksman had invented the term "antibiotic" in 1941.

Antibiotics today

Today, we have dozens of antibiotic drugs. Doctors prescribing them have to consider many factors. Some antibiotics are broad-spectrum, attacking many types of bacteria. Narrow-spectrum antibiotics kill only a few bacteria. Some types of bacteria become resistant to specific antibiotics, so others are tried against them. Some people are sensitive to one type of antibiotic, and so another type must be chosen for them. Antibiotics must be used carefully because bacteria can develop an immunity to them, and because people can become allergic to some antibiotics.

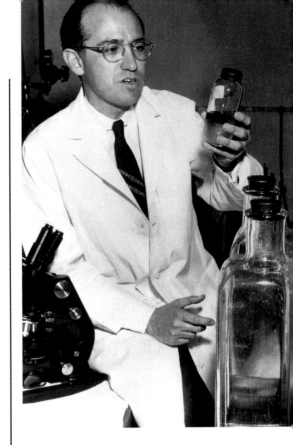

▲ Jonas Salk checks bottles of microbial growth in his University of Pittsburgh laboratory in 1955. He developed the Salk vaccine against the dreaded disease polio, saving thousands from death or crippling deformity.

Did You Know?

Malaria is one of the world's major diseases. For many years the most effective drug against it was quinine. This is a natural substance found in the bark of the cinchona tree, which grows in South America. Quinine was first purified in about 1630. Since about 1934, synthetic drugs, such as amodiaquine, have been used against malaria.

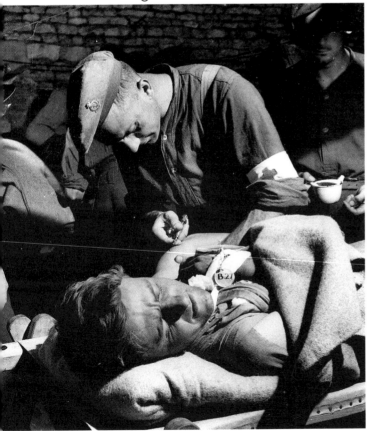

◀ Injured troops receive injections of antibiotics during World War II. Uncounted numbers of lives were saved by preventing infection of wounds.

Advances in Surgery

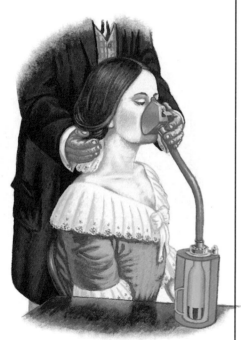

▲ This type of chloroform inhaler was used to put patients to sleep in the 1850s by John Snow, the first professional anesthetist in Great Britain.

William Morton publicly demonstrates ether as a general anesthetic at Massachusetts General Hospital in this painting by Robert Hinckley. ▶

During the early and mid-twentieth century, while patients were benefiting from the increasing numbers of drugs, there were also forward strides in surgery. These had been made possible by the discoveries of Lister and by the development of anesthesia in the previous century.

Anesthetics

Arabian doctors had used drugs to dull the senses during surgery. Two of these drugs were opium, from the opium poppy, and hyoscyamine, from plants such as henbane and deadly nightshade. Alcohol also put patients into a stupor. But for centuries, there was no good way to prevent the terrible pain of cutting during an operation. There was no way to put patients to sleep, so operations had to be performed very quickly.

In 1844, Connecticut dentist Horace Wells used the gas nitrous oxide to extract teeth painlessly from his patients. William Morton, also a dentist, used the fumes of liquid ether as an anesthetic. In 1846, he demonstrated this with a public tooth extraction. In October of

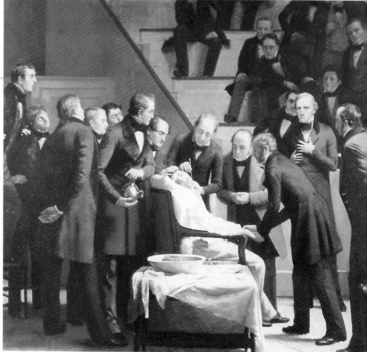

that year, he administered ether to a patient at Massachusetts General Hospital. Then Dr. John C. Warren painlessly removed a tumor from the man's jaw.

By 1847, chloroform was also being used. It was more controllable and had fewer bad effects. Since this time, anesthesia has become an important branch of medicine. The anesthetist is a vital part of the surgical team and has many techniques at his or her disposal. General anesthesia puts the patient to sleep. Local anesthesia deadens feeling in one part of the body.

Surgery and technology

Anesthesia allowed surgeons to take more time over their work. With the patient unconscious, the speed of the operation was less important. New and longer surgical operations could then be developed.

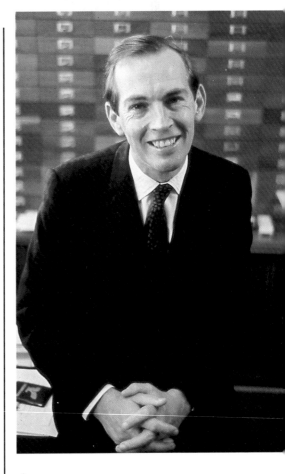

▲ Top: Pioneering surgeon Christiaan Barnard, operating on an anesthetized patient. Above: Dr. Barnard in Cape Town, South Africa, where he performed the world's first heart transplant in 1967.

X-rays and Radiology

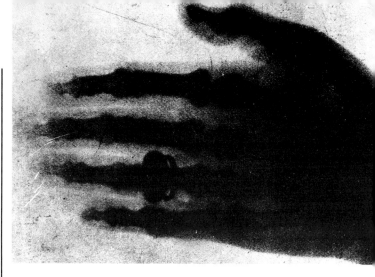

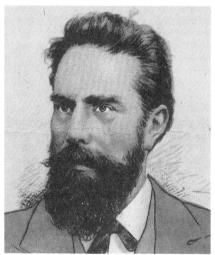

▲ Above: Wilhelm Röntgen won a Nobel Prize for his discovery of x-rays.

▲ Top right: Röntgen's x-ray of his wife's hand. The dense bones show up black. Modern x-rays show the dense parts white on a black background.

An x-ray clinic of the late 1800s. The risks of x-rays were not known then, so no one used protective screens or clothing. ▶

Did You Know?

The first patient to be helped by x-rays was Eddie McCarthy, an American from Dartmouth. In 1896, his broken arm was set using information from an x-ray photograph of his arm bones.

In 1895, physics professor Wilhelm Röntgen was experimenting with a new device called the vacuum tube, at Wurzburg in Germany. He discovered that it gave off invisible rays that could pass through less dense materials, like wood, but not through dense substances such as metals. He had little idea of the nature of the rays, so he called them x-rays.

Röntgen soon noticed that the rays passed through the body's flesh and muscle, but not through cartilage or bone. He took a picture of his wife's hand, in which the bones stood out clearly. It was the first x-ray image, or radiograph, of the body.

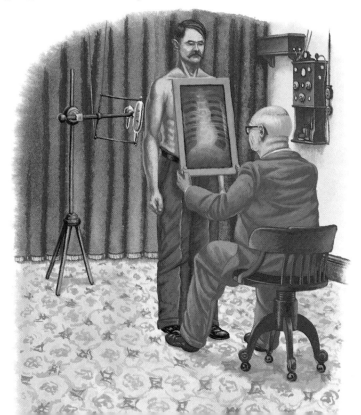

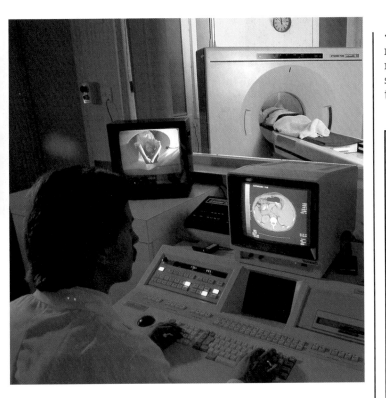

◀ A CAT scan in progress. The monitor screen in front of the radiographer shows a cross section through the abdomen of the patient.

Dangerous x-rays

Some early x-ray research workers suffered from skin ulcers, anemia, and certain types of cancers. These can also result from exposure to the naturally radioactive substances radium and polonium, discovered by Marie and Pierre Curie in 1899. It was shown that high doses of x-ray radiation harmed living tissues and brought on disease. Doctors turned this into an advantage by using carefully controlled doses of radiation to kill off diseased tissues such as cancers. This technique is known as radiotherapy.

The science of radiology

Doctors soon realized that these new x-rays could be used to show the inside of the body to locate foreign bodies or breaks in bones. At the turn of the century a technique was developed in which patients swallowed bismuth, a substance that shows up white on x-rays. A series of x-rays, taken as the bismuth moved through the digestive system, revealed any blockage or other problem.

In 1922, Jean Sicard and Jacques Forestier developed a similar technique for the lungs. An injection of a substance containing iodine showed up on the x-ray and outlined any abnormal areas in the air passages.

Since then, the branch of medicine known as radiology has made many advances. X-rays are linked with computers to produce CAT scans, images of entire sections of the body. Other techniques to form images from inside the body now include thermography (heat), echograms (sound waves), positron emission transaxial tomography (PETT), and nuclear magnetic resonance (NMR).

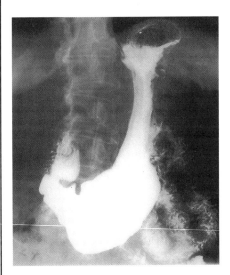

▲ An x-ray of the stomach, as a J-shaped bag. The patient had swallowed barium to produce the clear white outline. Behind, the bones of the spine show faintly.

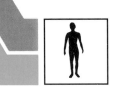

6: THE MEDICAL SYSTEM TODAY

Checkups and Tests

This youngster is getting a dental checkup. The dentist looks for early signs of tooth decay, gum disease, or other problems that are best treated before letting them get worse. ▶

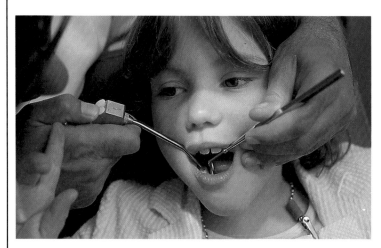

Medical science has developed many techniques that check for certain diseases or find early warning signs of trouble, even when the person has no symptoms. This is known as primary screening. We often say we are having a checkup. The earlier disease is discovered in a person, the earlier treatment can be started, with better chances of success.

Who to screen and what for
We cannot screen for every illness. Most people get better on their own from minor illnesses. Only certain more serious conditions, such as many cancers and heart problems, have early signs that can be detected rapidly and effectively. The test itself must not pose too many risks to the person being tested.

Screening may benefit people of a certain age who are most at risk from a certain illness, or one sex rather than another, or someone with a family history of the condition. So the screening is usually concentrated on a particular target group — those who are at risk.

The quality of life
One aim of medicine is to preserve and lengthen life. Another aim is to ease suffering. These two aims do not always go together. For example, a baby may be born badly deformed. The infant might need many operations to have a chance to survive. But it is not certain if treatment will succeed, or if it does, what sort of life the child would have.

An old, frail person may have a serious disease that could be curable — but only with extensive treatment that has many side effects.

In such cases the friends, relatives, doctors, and the patients themselves must decide very difficult questions. Is it worth giving treatment? If so, for how long? What are the chances of survival? Will the person be able to live a worthwhile life, able to enjoy happiness and contentment, without too much pain and suffering?

Diagnostic tests

A person with symptoms of illness visits the doctor. The doctor asks questions about the current problem and past health. This is known as taking a medical history.

The doctor may carry out diagnostic tests that can be done quickly in a clinic. For example, a urine sample could be tested with a chemically coated dipstick to check for abnormal urine contents.

If the problem cannot be identified, or if it needs further investigation, then other tests are scheduled. These range from taking a blood sample for later laboratory analysis, to visiting a hospital for an electrocardiogram or a scan.

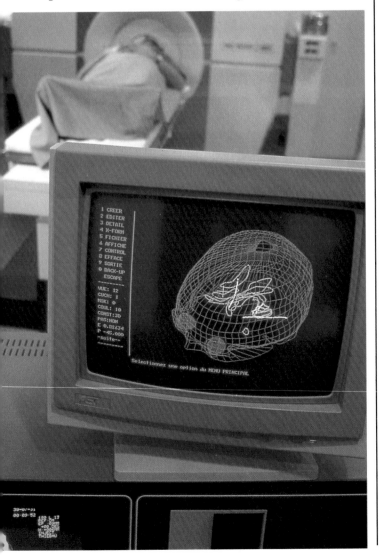

The Pap test

In 1928, the Greek-American scientist George Papanicolaou, working with a New York team, developed a test for cancers of the cervix — the neck of the uterus. A sample smear from the cervical lining could be checked under the microscope for early signs of disease, including precancerous cells. If detected early, there is an excellent chance of cure.

Today, the Pap test is widely used in many countries to screen for cervical disease. Generally, a woman has a test every year or so from the age of 25, or after childbirth, or if taking a contraceptive drug.

◀ The CAT scanner reveals a brain tumor, which the computer displays in green on its 3-D grid of the head. The tumor can be removed before it enlarges and causes more serious problems.

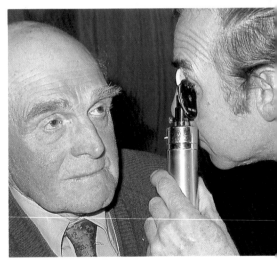

▲ An eye examination can also reveal general problems, such as high blood pressure, from the condition of the nerves and vessels visible in the retina at the back of the eye.

Electronic Eyes

Below: Thermography detects the temperatures of body parts. It can pick up "hot spots," such as abnormal growths. Below, right: Nuclear magnetic resonance (NMR) imaging shows the body's response to a strong magnetic field made by huge magnets. Bottom, right: The NMR scan shows soft tissues in detail — even the plum the patient is eating! ▼

ECGs and EEGs

As the heart pumps, and the muscles pull, and the brain thinks, they produce tiny bursts of electricity from muscular and nerve action. These bursts travel through the body. They can be detected on the skin by sensitive electrical equipment and shown visually for study by the doctor.

The ECG, or electrocardiograph, measures the electrical signals from the heart. These signals show up as wavy lines on paper or can be seen on a monitor screen. The pattern of the heart waves tells the doctor if the heart is enlarged, as in heart failure, or if parts of it are diseased or injured, as after a heart attack.

The EEG, or electroencephalograph, detects electrical signals from the brain. Their pattern can reveal abnormality or injury, as caused by a stroke, or a disease such as epilepsy. They can also detect the stages of sleep, and show which areas of the brain are involved when different senses are stimulated.

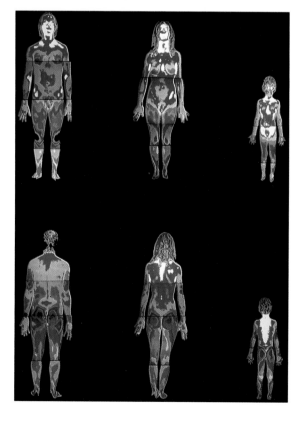

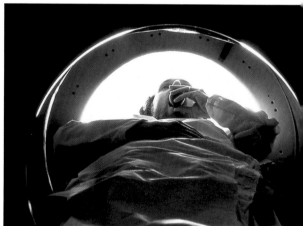

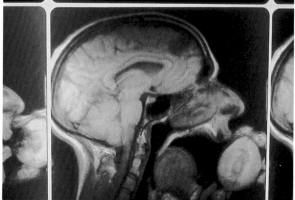

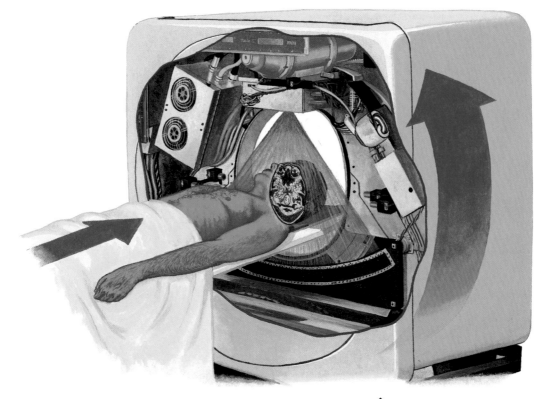

Seeing inside the body

The greatest area of medical progress over the last 30 years has been in imaging the structural details of the body's internal organs, without having to cut it open. X-rays were the first means of doing this. Today there are over a dozen techniques, and the images keep improving. Computers control the scanners, and they process, combine, and color the images so that doctors can see more clearly if there are any problems.

▲ The CAT scanner is like a rotating x-ray camera that revolves around the body in a giant drum. The x-rays are extremely weak and harmless, yet the combined image of a cross section through the body is very detailed.

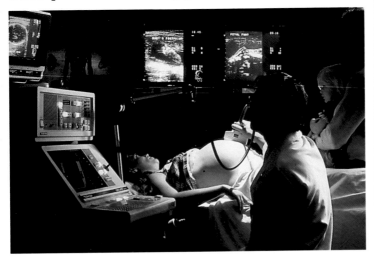

◄ This woman is having an ultrasound scan. High-pitched sound waves are beamed through her body. The computer processes the sound waves into an image that can be seen on a monitor screen. Ultrasound helps check that the developing baby is healthy.

41

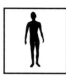

Drug Treatments

Developing a new drug takes years and costs millions. Only one from 1,000 to 10,000 of the possible drugs tried will make it through all the tests and be made available to patients. ▼

There are thousands of drugs. Some are extracted from natural sources like plants, but most are made in the laboratory. Each year sees dozens of new drugs.

Problems in prescribing

Prescribing the correct drug can be very complicated. First, it must be a drug that will act against the illness in question. Second, it must be the right dose for the person and the severity of the illness.

Besides this, there must be no contraindications. These are conditions or diseases that the patient has, or has had in the past, that could cause problems when the drug is given. For example, some drugs should not be given to people who have kidney disease or epilepsy.

Side effects

There are also side effects to think about. Sometimes the side effects of a powerful drug could be worse than letting the disease run its course. A few people are sensitive to certain drugs and should not have them prescribed. Also, a drug taken for a short time may interfere with one already being taken for a long-term condition, such as asthma or diabetes.

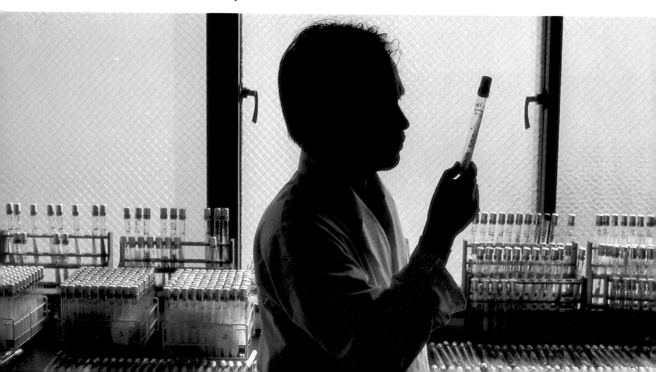

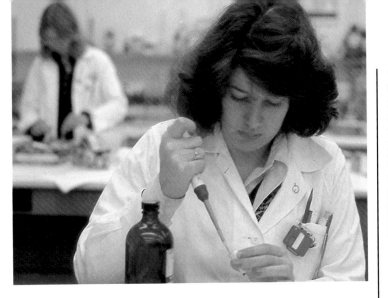

The way the body deals with a drug can give indications of illness. Samples of blood, urine, saliva, and other body fluids may be analyzed to find out how fast the drug is being broken down and into what end products.

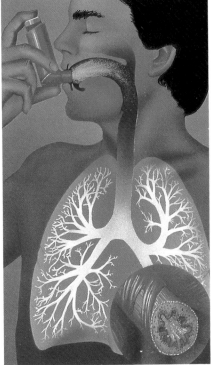

Learning from mistakes

New drugs have to be thoroughly tested on laboratory animals and on cells grown in the laboratory before the first trials are made on human volunteers. If a new drug passes all the tests, it goes into general use. Even then, problems with a drug often do not surface until years later, after thousands of people have taken it. In the 1950s, amphetamines were widely used as reducing pills. But people soon realized that their side effects and the problems of addiction far outweighed their usefulness. They were banned. Today, they are taken illegally as "speed," "pep pills," and "uppers."

Part of a drug's effectiveness depends on how and where it enters the body. Aerosol inhalers for controlling asthma deliver the drug as a fine mist into the airways where it is needed.

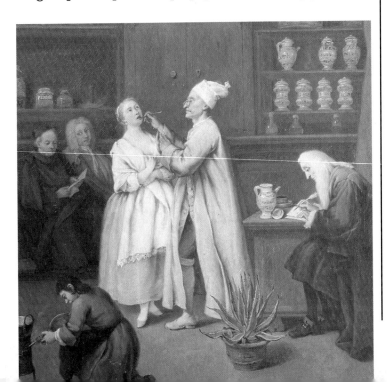

The old-time apothecary's shop was filled with minerals and processed parts of plants and animals. But the person who prescribed these items had to depend on memory. Today's doctors can refer to the extensive information available in books and by computers.

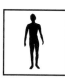

Surgery, Transplants, and Implants

Surgeons often specialize in one region of the body. A neurosurgeon focuses on the brain and nerves. A cardiac surgeon operates on the heart and major blood vessels. An orthopedic surgeon deals with bones and joints.

Any complicated operation is usually performed by a surgical team. There are the chief and assistant surgeons, the anesthetist, the nursing staff, and specialists handling complex machinery, such as heart-lung machines and x-ray equipment.

Transplants

A transplanted part is taken from one person, the donor, and put into the body of another, the recipient. The donor may be a living person, such as a relative who donates a kidney to a family member with kidney failure. Or the donor may have died, usually as the result of an accident such as a car crash. The donor, or the nearest relative of a dead person, must give permission for the parts to be used for transplants.

A heart transplant was news in the 1970s. In the 1980s, it became more common. Other

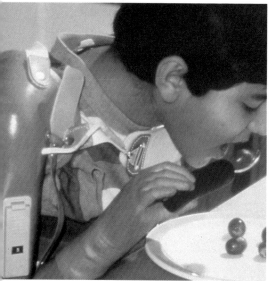

▲ This boy is learning to use his new myoelectric limb, a device that replaces a limb lost through accident or disease. Tiny sensors on the skin of the stump detect electrical signals from muscles inside. These are amplified and sent to electric motors and other parts that move the arm.

A Starr-Edwards heart valve (inset) and an x-ray image of it in position in a living heart. ▶

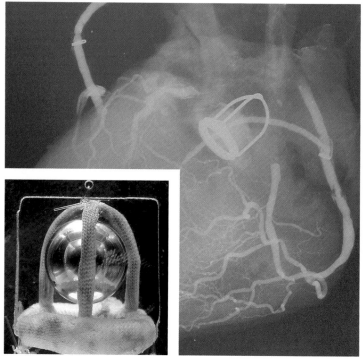

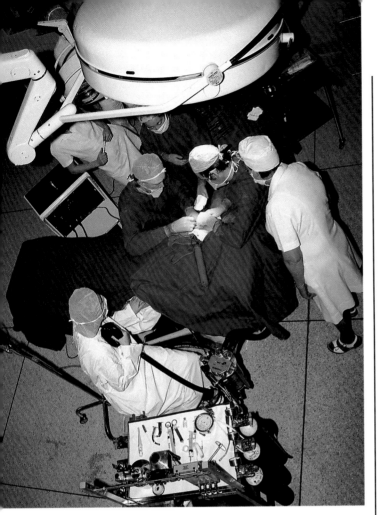

Transplants and implants: ▼

1. Metal plate
2. Plastic eye
3. Artificial ear
4. Bridge anchor
5. Jaw
6. Teeth
7. Larynx
8. Lung
9. Arm
10. Pacemaker
11. Valve
12. Heart
13. Breast implant
14. Shoulder joint
15. Elbow joint
16. Wrist joint
17. Knuckles
18. Liver
19. Kidney
20. Pancreas
21. Insulin pump
22. Hip joint
23. Metal thighbone
24. Knee
25. Metal shin
26. Leg

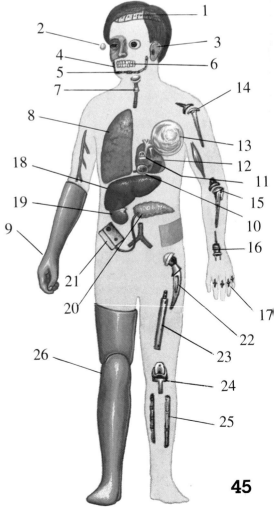

transplanted parts include the heart and lungs together as a unit, liver, kidney, pancreas, bone marrow, cornea, larynx (voice box), trachea (windpipe), and, of course, blood in a blood transfusion.

A major problem is that the recipient's body fights against the transplant as if it were a foreign invader. In the 1980s, new types of immunosuppressive drugs were developed. These inhibit the defending immune system, so that there is less chance of the patient's body rejecting the transplant.

Implants

Artificial body parts, such as false teeth, have been used for centuries. But over the past 40 years, many new spare parts have been developed. They need to be made of substances that do the job and that the body will not reject, such as special metals and plastics.

45

Treating the Mind

Modern life's many stresses, such as overwork and worries about jobs and personal relations, can place a great strain on a person's mental health. Such stresses in someone who already has mental burdens due, for example, to a poor self-image or setting goals that may be unrealistic, can result in serious emotional conflicts. If not treated, these conflicts could lead to mental illness. ▶

The ancient doctors of China, Greece, and India knew that some illnesses did not involve physical problems that might have symptoms such as a growth or a swelling. These illnesses seemed to be based in people's minds. The only signs were in the way people behaved, how they handled their emotions, and what reactions they showed. Early views of mental illness were often linked to magic, superstition, and being possessed by evil spirits.

For centuries during the Middle Ages, people with mental illnesses were locked away in asylums and forgotten. In many asylums, the conditions were dreadful. There was little hope of receiving treatment or being freed. The public paid to come and see the "mad people," taunting them into an outburst.

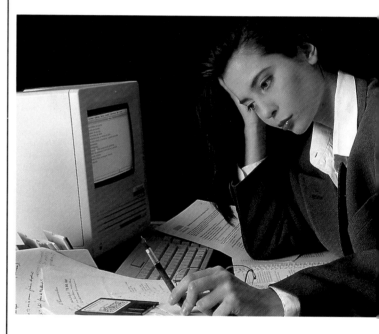

The beginnings of psychiatry

In the late 1800s and early 1900s, some doctors became interested in mental illness. One of the first who tried to explain such illnesses and devise treatments was a physician from Vienna, Sigmund Freud. He founded several areas of psychology — the scientific study of how the mind works, and why we act and behave as we do.

Freud was also involved in the early stages of psychiatry — the study, diagnosis, and treatment of mental illnesses. He was the first to treat patients with psychoanalysis.

Several of Freud's fellow doctors eventually disagreed with him, and they left to establish their own schools of psychology. Alfred Adler, an Austrian, departed in 1911. Carl Jung, the first president of the International Psychoanalytic Association, left in 1913. Both men made major contributions to modern psychiatry — a branch of medicine.

Psychiatrists are physicians who specialize in mental illness. Psychologists study how people think and behave, but they do not treat mental illness. Research into the workings of the brain indicates that some kinds of mental illness may have a physical basis.

Illness of the mind

Most people cope with life's ups and downs. Although they are sometimes very sad, or worried, they shrug off such feelings and behave again in a reasonable and sensible way.

In mental illness, the person's mind and thinking become abnormal. He or she cannot cope with daily life and will show strange behavior, odd moods, and irrational reactions.

Mental illnesses are often difficult to identify and explain because human behavior is so complicated and variable. Also, what people regard as "normal behavior" varies from place to place and from one time to another.

In general, if the illness is less severe, and the person realizes that there is a problem, the person has what is called a neurosis. Examples are bouts of severe depression, or the compulsion to wash hands after touching any object. But in a psychosis, the person loses touch with reality and does not realize that there is something wrong.

◀ Sigmund Freud, founder of psychoanalysis. He thought that our unconscious thoughts reveal our worries and anxieties through our dreams. By analyzing these unconscious thoughts, Freud believed that we could overcome our problems.

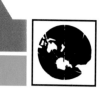

China and the Far East

Chinese medicine

Chinese medical care today still relies on the past traditions called *Chung-i*. It also uses methods from India combined with the new technologies and drugs from the West.

There is a strong belief in China that health in the body is based on the harmony of opposing forces. These forces are called yin and yang. Illness happens when the forces are out of balance, and the traditional treatments use healing energies that work to restore the balance of the yin and yang. Other forms of treatment used in China are acupuncture, massage, and special healing exercises.

Barefoot doctors

China's population is so great that one-fifth of the people of the world live in that one country. This means there is a lack of funds to provide enough fully trained doctors. Part-time health workers, called "barefoot doctors," are trained for about six months in traditional and Western medicine. They concentrate on problems such as coughs, colds, lack of

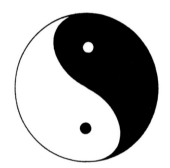

▲ The traditional Chinese symbol of balance in a healthy body. These opposing forces are called yin (which is cool and "female") and yang (hot and "male"). Here these forces are represented by the dark and light colors.

Traditional remedies on display in a street market in southern China. Many traders have extensive knowledge of what remedy is suitable for what disease, and how to prepare it. ▶

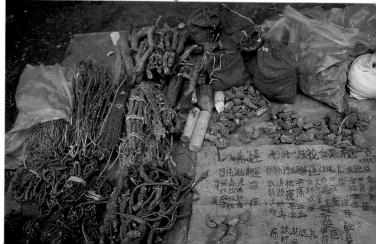

healthy food, and infection due to poor sanitation. They also give advice about pregnancy and childbirth, child care, preventing illness, and birth control. They have been very successful, and there are now over 1,300,000 of these community health workers.

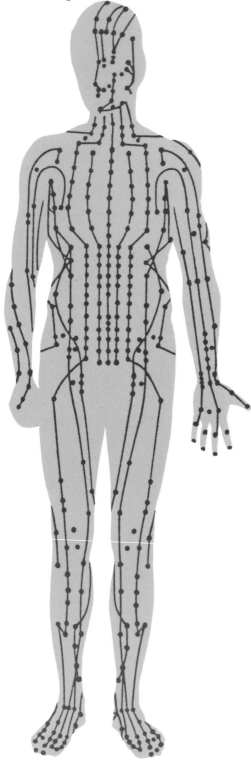

◀ The acupuncture channels, or meridians, carry *chi* energy through the body. Needles in the insertion points either speed or slow this energy flow.

Inserting acupuncture needles on a patient's head. In China and Japan, acupuncture is a widespread form of treatment. ▼

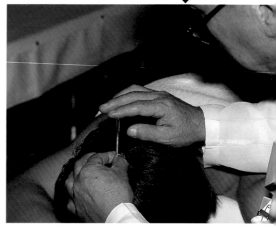

India and the Middle East

Health workers give advice ▶
about family planning methods.
This is part of India's campaign
to slow the increase in the
population.

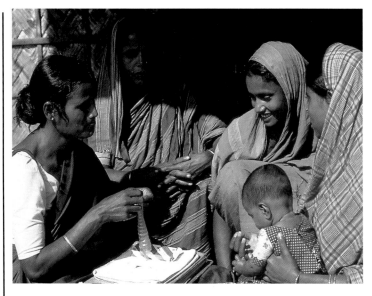

The traditional medicine of India, *ayurveda*,
goes back over 3,000 years. It is based on centuries of experience with herbs and other medicinal substances. Practitioners in over 14,000
dispensaries in India advise patients and supply traditional cures.

   Most Indian doctors are trained in both traditional and Western medicine. However, in
many places, especially in cities, traditional
techniques are regarded less highly, and
many doctors practice the kind of medicine we
are familiar with in the West.

Medical facts: India

- Life expectancy is 58 years.

- Infant mortality is around 110
deaths for every 1,000 babies.

- Birth control is seen as the
chief means of reducing the
population. Too many people
lead to shortages in food
supplies, water and sanitation
systems, and health services.

- There is one qualified doctor
for every 3,600 people.

- There is one hospital bed for
every 1,600 people.

Shantytowns, such as this one in
India, encourage the spread of
diseases. Flies carry germs from
the open sewers onto food, and the
drinking water is contaminated. ▶

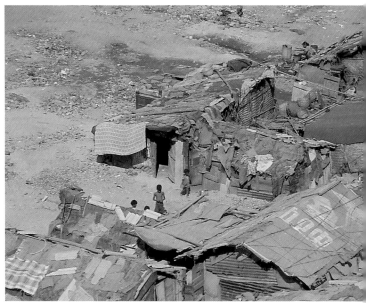

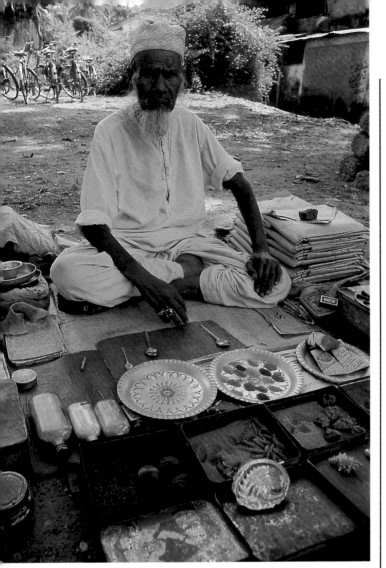

◀ A street medical trader in Karwar, in southern India. In areas where there are no officially qualified doctors, traditional traders give advice and supply medicines.

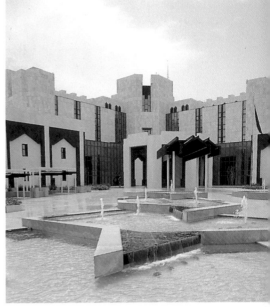

▲ The King Khalid Eye Hospital in Saudi Arabia. This oil-rich nation uses its wealth to bring about improved health care and modern medical facilities.

This herb, rauwolfia, has been used for more than 2,000 years in India. Its roots contain the drug reserpine, which helps soothe the brain and nervous system. It also calms the heart and lowers blood pressure. ▼

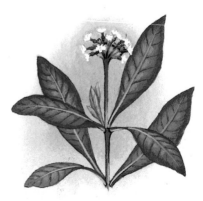

In Pakistan, traditional medicine is known as *unani-tibb*. It is carried out by doctors who are trained at medical schools and who also study Western methods.

Rich and poor

The Middle East is another area with a long tradition of healing. Today, it is a region of contrasts. Some countries have become rich from selling oil and have bought expertise and up-to-date equipment from the West. Neighboring poor countries, without oil, struggle to provide clean water and proper sewage disposal in attempts to prevent diseases such as cholera and dysentery. They also lack money to teach their people about basic hygiene, which can prevent illnesses.

Africa

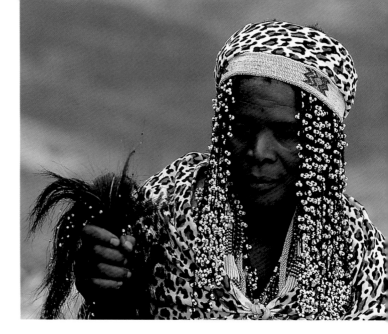

A traditional diviner from ▶ southern Africa. She holds a special object which helps her to concentrate and direct her spiritual powers.

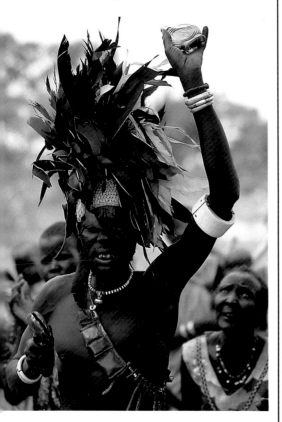

▲ A *binjar*, or traditional healer, from southern Sudan, holding a bottle of medicine during a healing ceremony.

Healing by the spirits

The traditional medicine of many African groups is centered on the healer — a person with special powers. This is usually a man, who has been chosen early in life and served a long period of training with his predecessor. He learns how to make and use medicines and how to make contact with the spirit world during healing ceremonies. The spirits pass their powers through him, and so he is able to cure the sick. Over 90% of the medicines used in this type of healing come from plants.

These traditional treatments are passed on by word of mouth, so knowledge about them is in danger of disappearing as societies adopt Western ways. Traditional healers are now part of the state medical system in some countries, such as Zimbabwe.

Hunger and malnutrition

In Africa, the main causes of disease are lack of food, poverty, and poor sanitation. Not enough food means that people develop malnutrition and become ill more easily. Enough food for everyone can result in better health.

The main aims of the health services are to control tropical diseases caused by parasites, such as malaria; to grow enough food for everyone to have a healthy diet; to wipe out

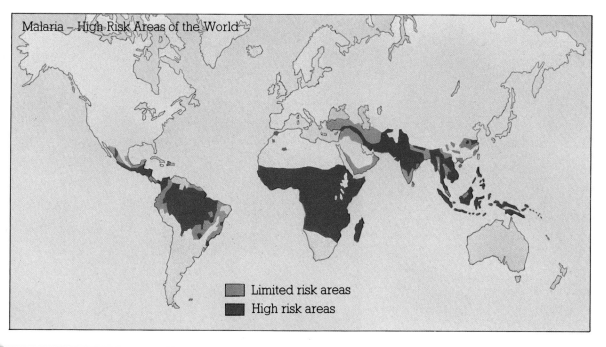

Malaria – High Risk Areas of the World

Limited risk areas
High risk areas

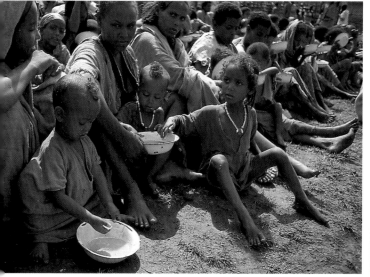

▲ Malaria is still one of the world's most serious health problems.

◀ These children from famine-stricken Ethiopia have a poor diet that makes them more likely to develop illnesses. Medical care cannot replace the basic human need for food.

diseases, using drugs donated by wealthier countries; and to immunize more children against the common infections.

Where you are and who you are

In Africa, as in many regions, medicine varies even within a country. Are there health facilities in your area, and if there are, can you use them? You might be kept from doing so because of your cultural or ethnic group, or your lack of money or health insurance.

Medical facts: Kenya

- Life expectancy for women is about 61 years, and for men it is 57 years.

- Infant mortality is less than 50 deaths for every 1,000 babies.

- There is one qualified doctor for every 10,000 people.

- There is one hospital bed for every 1,000 people.

The Americas

This man from Ecuador grows medicinal herbs in his garden, 12,000 feet (3,700 m) high in the Andes. In such remote areas, people rely on themselves for medicines. ▶

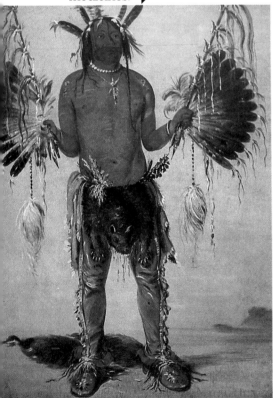

▲ The Mandan medicine man, Mah-To-He-Ha ("Old Bear"), painted by the famous North American artist George Catlin in 1832.

The native peoples of North, Central, and South America had their own traditional types of medicine. Today, traditional medicine is still used in remote areas, such as the Amazon rain forest and the Andes. But in most other places, modern Western-style medicine has taken over.

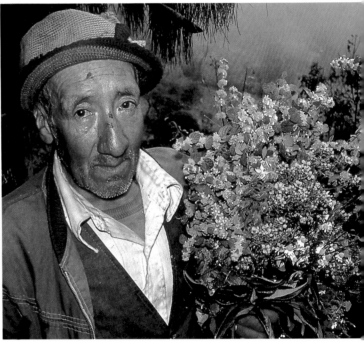

North American Indians

Many Indian groups believe that illness is due to forces from the spirit world, especially those connected with animals, plants, and nature. Their view of medicine is tied in with their living with the natural world and trying to conserve it, rather than destroy it. For example, the spirits might be displeased because an animal had been killed at the wrong time, and so the spirits would bring the curse of illness.

When a North American Indian became ill, he or she consulted the group's herbalist. If medicinal herbs did not work, then a spirit healer might be called in to try to find the cause through divining.

The spirit healer would smoke, sniff, or chew on certain drug-containing plants, and enter a

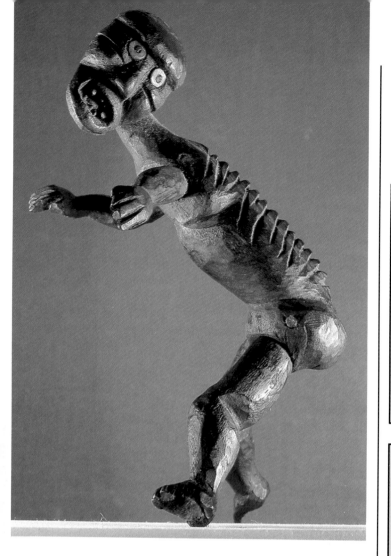

◀ In some Inuit groups of North America, small figures and statues are made as offerings to the spirits for a long and healthy life. But this figure, called a *tupilaq*, is intended to bring harm to others!

Medical facts: Brazil

- Life expectancy for women is about 67 years, and for men around 62 years.

- Infant mortality is less than 70 deaths for every 1,000 babies.

- There is one qualified hospital doctor for every 2,300 people.

- There is one hospital bed for every 280 people.

Medical facts: Bolivia

- Life expectancy is 50 years.

- Infant mortality is 120 deaths for every 1,000 babies.

trance to communicate with the spirits. In this drug-induced state, the healer supposedly had special healing powers.

South American Indians

The Indians of South America also rely mainly on medicinal plants for healing. One famous group is the Kallawaya, from Bolivia. In the Aymara language, their name means "carrying medicine on the shoulder." They carry bags of dried herbs with them as they travel around, diagnosing and treating illnesses and holding curing ceremonies.

In many cultures, such as some Indian groups, knowing of medicine and healing gives the doctor power and influence in the community. So he keeps his knowledge and skills as well-guarded secrets.

Did You Know?

Some of the greatest epidemics have been caused by mild illnesses introduced to a new group of people, who have no resistance. During the invasion of Mexico by Hernando Cortes in 1520, hundreds of thousands of Mexican Indians died from diseases, such as smallpox and measles, that were brought by the invaders. Some experts estimate that in the 100 years following the European invasion of the Americas, over 50 million American Indians perished from such diseases.

8: MEDICINE IN THE FUTURE

The Coming Challenges

Medicine continues to face many challenges. Some challenges, like malaria, have probably been around since history began. Others, such as AIDS, are recent.

Environmental causes of illness

Each year, about six million people in the world develop cancers. In these diseases, body cells suddenly go out of control. They fail to do their usual jobs. They begin to multiply and form growths, and they spread through the body.

For many years, the causes of cancers were a mystery. But more and more cancers are being linked with our environment. Certain chemicals, such as dioxin, tobacco smoke, and asbestos, can trigger cancers in the body. So can the wrong types of food, too much radiation, and many other factors.

New diseases

In the early 1980s, a new disease was recognized, first in the United States and then in

Smallpox facts

Smallpox has probably killed and disfigured more people than any other disease. In the 1700s alone, it killed about 60 million people. In 1967, the World Health Organization began a campaign to wipe out this disease by vaccination and other measures. In 1979, the world officially became free of smallpox.

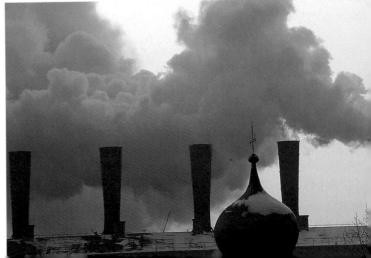

Factory chimneys polluting the air. In years to come, we may discover that some of the air pollutants we pour into the atmosphere today cause slowly developing illnesses. Clean air, like good food and pure water, is necessary for health. ▶

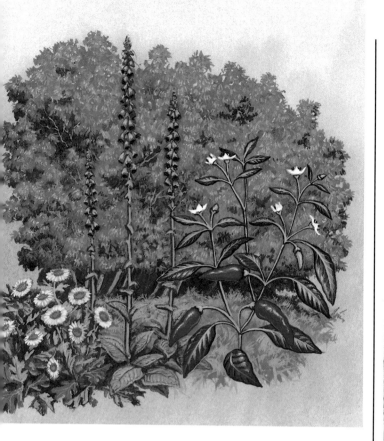

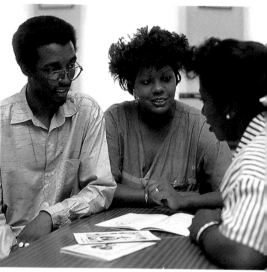

◀ The foxglove flower (center) has been used for centuries as a medicinal plant. Its various medical drug ingredients, such as digitalis, digoxin, and digitoxin, help the heart beat slower and more strongly. In the 1700s, Dr. William Withering of England was the first to prescribe digitalis for some of his heart patients.

▲ Certain diseases tend to run in families or are more common in some ethnic groups. A genetic counselor is a medical specialist who can advise on the risks of children being affected.

other countries. The disease attacked the body's immune system. This is our body's ability to resist disease. Without it, we cannot fight against illness. The disease was named acquired immune deficiency syndrome (AIDS). The cause was found to be human immunodeficiency virus (HIV).

At the end of the 1980s, the World Health Organization estimated that 600,000 people around the world suffered from AIDS. But millions more have the virus, especially in Africa, and they will eventually develop the disease. Doctors say this disease is incurable.

Millions of dollars have been spent on research into AIDS. So far, this has resulted in new knowledge of the workings of the human immune system. We are still learning about this unusual virus. Many steps have been taken toward effective drug treatments and vaccines for this disease. Whether or not a cure is found for AIDS, people with other diseases will benefit from this research.

Success story

Many cancers are now being treated more successfully. This is due to earlier detection and to treatments combining drugs, radiotherapy, and surgery. For example, acute lymphatic leukemia is a blood cancer of children. In the late 1950s, only one patient in 25 was cured. By the late 1970s, it was one in two. During this same period, the cure rate for Hodgkin's disease, a cancer of the lymph glands, also improved from two patients in five to four in five.

MEDICINE IN THE FUTURE

Healing the World

In the future, our medicine of today will be part of history. People may look back at our times and wonder: Why did we have to cut people open to cure them? Why did we struggle so hard to understand mental illness? And most of all, why were millions of people in some parts of the world dying of hunger, yet in other parts of the world, great amounts of money were being spent on drugs and surgery for just a few people?

Romanian children infected with AIDS. These children do not have access to expensive hospitals, equipment, the latest technology, and the best medicine. They have only the barest medical care. ▶

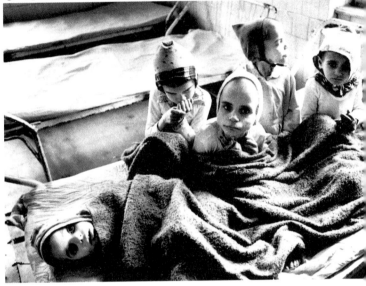

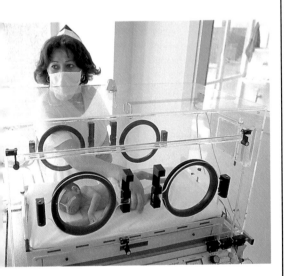

▲ In contrast to the Romanian children, this newborn British baby is being looked after with great care, using an incubator and other specialized equipment.

Basic needs
Better health for millions of people throughout the world depends, not on better medical care, but on fulfilling basic human needs. People need enough good food, clean water, sanitation, and good living conditions. These challenges for society as a whole are complicated by wars, religions, and politics.

Immunization programs
The elimination of smallpox shows that we can succeed in ridding the world of a disease. Immunization programs are one of the most effective ways of doing this. But programs such as this require great amounts of money for health workers, vaccines, equipment, and the spread of information. Currently, more money is being spent to develop weapons.

Prevention is better than cure

Slowly, people, especially those in rich countries, are realizing that they can, and should,
prevent illness by taking better care of themselves. This means eating nutritious food,
avoiding becoming overweight, and exercising, among other things. It involves cleaning
up our environment and reducing our use of
dangerous and polluting chemicals.

Medicine for all?

Today, as in the past, medicine is connected
with people's attitudes toward health and
illness and to their traditions and beliefs.
Medical progress relies on the research and
discoveries made by scientists. It also depends on how much money we are willing to
spend for this research and for medical care.
This is not a decision for doctors and patients
alone, but a question for all of society.

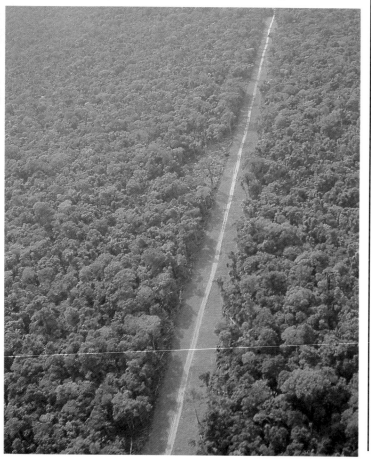

Holistic health

Modern Western-style medicine
tends to treat just a particular
symptom, or a part of the body.
It does not take into account the
whole person, including the
person's mind, emotions, out-
look, attitude, and feelings
toward life. Holistic medicine
has this approach, and it has
become more popular. Some
experts predict that it will be a
guiding force in the future of
medical care.

◀ A strip cleared through the
Amazon rain forest to make room
for a new highway. Many of our
medicines have come from
nature. Yet in many places, such
as here in Brazil, people are
destroying plants and animals
before they can be investigated
for their medicinal properties.

Glossary

AIDS: A short way of saying acquired immune deficiency syndrome. This disease attacks the body's ability to fight infections. Because of this, common diseases can become deadly in people who have AIDS.

Amphetamines: Drugs, made in laboratories, that can stimulate the body.

Anatomist: A person who studies the structures of the body.

Anatomy: The structures of the human body, such as nerves, muscles, bones, and so on.

Anemia: A blood disease in which there are not enough red blood cells, or the red cells are too small, or the red cells do not have enough hemoglobin — a substance that carries oxygen throughout the body. People who have anemia tire out quickly and cannot fight off infections easily.

Anesthesia: Numbness, or lack of feeling, caused by a drug. An anesthetic is used to keep a person from feeling pain during surgery. A general anesthetic causes the person to become unconscious.

Anthrax: A disease that affects humans and cattle. It involves spots, sores, and lung infection. Anthrax can be carried on hides and furs that are poorly prepared.

Antibiotic: A substance, originally from mold, that fights infection by bacteria.

Antiseptic: A chemical substance that kills or disables bacteria, fungi, or viruses.

Arteries: Tubes that carry blood from the heart to all parts of the body.

Asbestos: A mineral once used in insulation, fireproofing, and in many other ways. It can cause cancer in humans.

Asthma: A disease of the lungs that causes periodic difficulty in breathing.

Bacteria: One-celled living things visible only under a microscope. Some kinds of bacteria can cause infections in plants or animals.

Bacteriology: The study of bacteria.

Blood vessels: The tubes that carry blood around the body. They consist of arteries, capillaries, and veins.

Capillaries: The tiniest blood vessels, visible only under a microscope. They are the connection between the arteries and veins.

Cell: The smallest living unit. Some cells, like a bacterium, can live independently. Other living things are made up of many cells.

Cellular pathology: The study of the changes that take place in cells when they become abnormal in some way because of infection or other forms of disease.

Chiropractor: A health care professional who treats disease by relieving pressure on nerves and muscles that is caused by joints and bones that have moved slightly out of line.

Chloroform: A gas that can cause anesthesia. At one time, chloroform was used in medicine, but now we use better and safer anesthetics.

Cholera: A disease of the intestines that causes constant diarrhea. It is caused by bacteria and spread by unclean water and food.

Contaminated: Spoiled or tainted as a result of containing harmful chemicals or disease-causing microbes in or on another substance.

Culture: In bacteriology, the growing of bacterial or other microbes in the laboratory in order to study them. Cultures can be grown on a jelly-like substance in shallow plates called petri dishes, or in a broth in bottles. This word can also refer to the physical and spiritual way of life of a particular group of people.

Dark Ages: Another name for the Middle Ages, or the medieval period, in European history. It lasted from about the fifth century to the fourteenth century. During this time there was little progress in the arts, sciences, and medicine.

Diabetes: A short way of saying *diabetes mellitus*. This disease is caused by a shortage of the hormone insulin, and this leads to excess sugar in the blood.

Diagnosis: The finding out of which disease or condition a sick person has.

Dioxins: Very poisonous substances formed when some kinds of plastics and other substances are manufactured.

Diphtheria: An infectious disease in which a person's throat is obstructed by a thick growth. This blocks the air passage, interferes with breathing, and can cause death.

Dispensary: A place where drugs and other medicines are given to patients.

Diviner: A person said to have the ability to use supernatural means to find water, ores, or the cause of sickness.

Dysentery: An intestinal infection by bacteria or other organisms that involves digestive upset, pains, and diarrhea.

Embryology: The study of the growth and development of babies in the mother's uterus before they are born.

Epidemic: The rapid spread of disease through a large number of people in an area. When the area is huge, the epidemic is a pandemic.

Epilepsy: A disease of the nervous system that can cause convulsions.

Fallopian tubes: The tubes through which eggs from female mammals travel to the uterus, or womb. They are also called oviducts.

Fermenting: The process of a substance breaking down to simpler substances over time. This is caused by microbes.

Gout: A disease that causes some joints of the body to swell up from time to time so that movement is difficult and painful.

Herbalist: A person who uses plants and herbs as medicines to treat some illnesses.

Hydraulic: Worked by liquids under pressure. The brakes of a car and the digging arm of a backhoe are examples of hydraulic mechanisms.

Immune: To be protected from catching an infection.

Immunization: Making the body build up protection against a particular disease by giving the person a small amount of a disease-causing microbe.

Immunosuppressive: A word describing the action of certain drugs in blocking the full activity of the body's immune system.

Implant: A human-made device that replaces a natural body part that had to be removed because of disease or damage.

Industrial Revolution: The time in Europe and North America when people changed from making things by hand to making them by machines in factories. This shift took place from about 1750 to 1850.

Iodine: A chemical element often used as an antiseptic when made into a solution.

Lymph glands: Structures in the body that produce lymph, the fluid part of blood.

Malaria: A disease caused by a one-celled parasite of the red blood cells. The female of a type of mosquito can pass on this disease through a bite. A person with malaria has periods of chills and fever.

Mental illness: An illness of the mind that affects a person's behavior, emotions, and reactions to persons and events.

Microbes: Small organisms, such as bacteria, fungi, and protists, that can be seen only under a microscope.

Microbiologist: A person who studies microscopic organisms, such as bacteria and fungi.

Microstructures: Very small patterns of cells that can be seen only under a microscope.

Neanderthal: A type of human that lived from about 120,000 to 40,000 years ago from western Europe to central Asia. Neanderthals were shorter and stockier than people of today. They used fire and made tools.

Nobel Prize: One of several prizes in different categories that are awarded yearly by the Nobel Foundation in Stockholm. The awards were established by Alfred Nobel, a Swedish industrialist who invented dynamite. The prizes have been awarded since 1901.

Nutrient jelly: A jelly that contains nutrients and is used in laboratories to grow some types of organisms.

Osteopath: A health professional who treats muscle pain, swollen joints, and similar problems with manipulation and massage.

Papyrus: A type of writing paper used by ancient Egyptians. Papyrus was made from reeds that grew in the Nile River.

Parasite: Animal or plant organisms that live on or in other animals, humans, or plants, using the larger animal, human, or plant for food and as a home. This can cause illness to the larger organism.

Pathology: The study of how disease affects the human body.

Physiology: The study of the way living things and their parts work.

Psychiatry: A branch of medicine that studies and treats mental illnesses.

Radiation: Energy in the form of invisible rays or particles that can damage living tissues. X-rays are one kind of radiation.

Renaissance: A period of European history from the early fourteenth to the late sixteenth century. The Renaissance marks the change from the Middle Ages to the modern era. During this period, there was a revival in the arts, literature, and sciences.

Sperm: Sex cells made by the male that fertilize the eggs made by the female so that they develop into babies.

Stupor: A dullness of the mind or body that causes a person to act and think slowly or in a confused manner.

Symptoms: The features of an illness that the person with that sickness notices.

Tissues: A group of cells working together to do a particular job in the body. The entire body is made up of different kinds of tissues.

Transplant: An organ or other human part that replaces a part of a person that has been damaged or diseased.

Tuberculosis: A bacterial infection, mainly of the lungs, causing fever, coughing, and weakened bodily condition. It is also called TB. Tuberculosis can cause death if untreated.

Veins: Tubes that collect blood from the arteries and carry it back to the heart.

Virus: The smallest organism that can live inside plants and animals. It cannot be seen under a microscope. Some viruses cause disease in plants, animals, and humans.

Index

A **boldface** number shows that the entry is illustrated on that page. The same page often has text about the entry, too.

Papanicolaou, George (American cellular pathologist) 39
Paracelsus (German-Swiss physician) **22**, 23
Paré, Ambroise (Andre) (French physician) **23**
Pasteur, Louis (French chemist) **26**
pathology 23, 26
  cellular 29
pediatricians 9
penicillin 11, **32**
Persia, famous physicians of 17
PETT (*see* positron emission transaxial tomography)
phlegm 15
physical therapists 5
physiology 21, 23
plague, bubonic 16, 17
polio 33
poppy sap 11 (*see also* opium)
positron emission transaxial tomography (PETT) 37
pregnancy 9, **16**, **41**, 49
preventive medicine 6-7, 14, 59
psychology and psychiatry **30**, 31, **46-47**
psychoses 47
pulse rate 8, 21

qualities of life, the four ancient 15
quality of life and modern medical treatment 38
quinine 25, 33

radiology **36-37**
radiotherapy 37
Ramazzini, Bernardino (Italian physician) 22
rauwolfia **51**
Reed, Walter (American physician) 30, **31**
religion and medicine 10, 11, 13, 14, **17**, **18**-19 (*see also* African medicine, American Indian medicine, Chinese medicine, Egyptian medicine, ancient, Greek medicine, ancient, India, medicine of, *and* Roman medicine, ancient)
Renaissance, medicine in the **20**-21, 22
Rhazes (Persian physician) 17
Roman medicine, ancient **12-13**
Röntgen, Wilhelm (German physicist) **36**

saints as healers **17**
Salk, Jonas (American microbiologist) **33**
Salvarsan 31
Sanctorius, Santorio (Italian physician) 21
scans **37**, **39**, **40-41**
scientific methods in medicine, beginnings of 12, **22-29**
screening **38-39**
side effects of drugs 42
smallpox 26, 55, 56, 58
Smith papyrus 11
smoking 6, **7**
Snow, John (British anesthetist) 34
South American Indian medicine 55
specialists 9, 44, **45**
suicide 4
Sumatra, medicine in **6**
suntan **4**
superstition (*see* African medicine, American Indian medicine, Chinese medicine, Egyptian medicine, ancient, Greek medicine, ancient, India, medicine of, *and* Roman medicine, ancient)
Surgeon Dentist, or Treatise of the Teeth, The 25
surgery 7, **23**, 34, **35**
  amputation **5**
surgical instruments **10-11**, 17, **45**
Susruta (Indian physician) 17
Sydenham, Thomas (English physician) 24, **25**

tannic acid 11
temperature, body 21, 25, **40**
thermography 37, **40**
transplants and implants **44-45**
trepanning 10-**11**
tuberculosis (TB) 5, 27
tupilaq (Inuit figurine) **55**

ultrasound scans **41**
unani-tibb (Pakistani traditional medicine) 51
United Nations 5
United States, medicine in the **6**-7, 8
Universa Medicina 23

vaccination 26, 33 (*see also* immunization)
Vesalius, Andreas (Belgian physician) **21**

Virchow, Rudolf (Prussian pathologist) 29
von Behring, Emil (German bacteriologist) 31

Waksman, Selman (American microbiologist) 33
Wells, Horace (American dentist) 34
WHO (World Health Organization) 5, 56, 57
Withering, William (English physician) 57
"wonder drugs" 7, 32-**33**

x-rays 9, **36-37**

yellow fever 30, 31
yin and yang **48**